Herbs to

Herbal First Aid Handbook

For:

* Home
* Travel
* Wilderness Survival
* Outdoor Sports
* When the Emergency Arises

Kurt King, M.H.

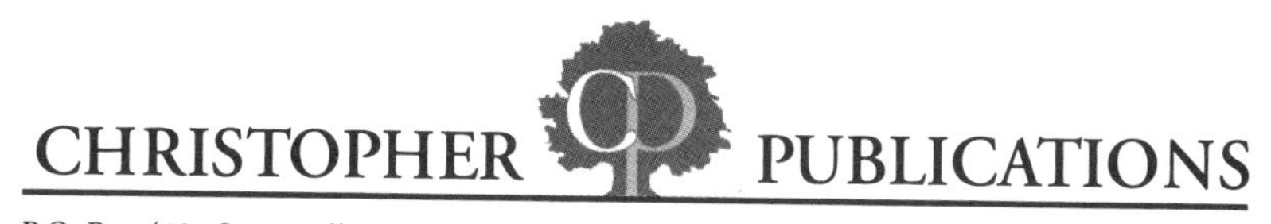

P.O. Box 412 · Springville, Utah 84663 1-888-489-0155 · www.christopherpublications.com

Christopher Publications, Inc. offers many books, CD's and DVD's to educate about the uses of herbs and natural healing, which are available for retail and wholesale purchase.

For more information, please contact:
www.christopherpublications.com
Christopher Publications, Inc.
P.O. Box 412
Springville UT 84663
1-888-489-0155

Project Editor
Janae King, M.H.

Reprinted 2010 and 2022

Printed in the U.S.A.
Signature Book Printing
sbpbooks.com

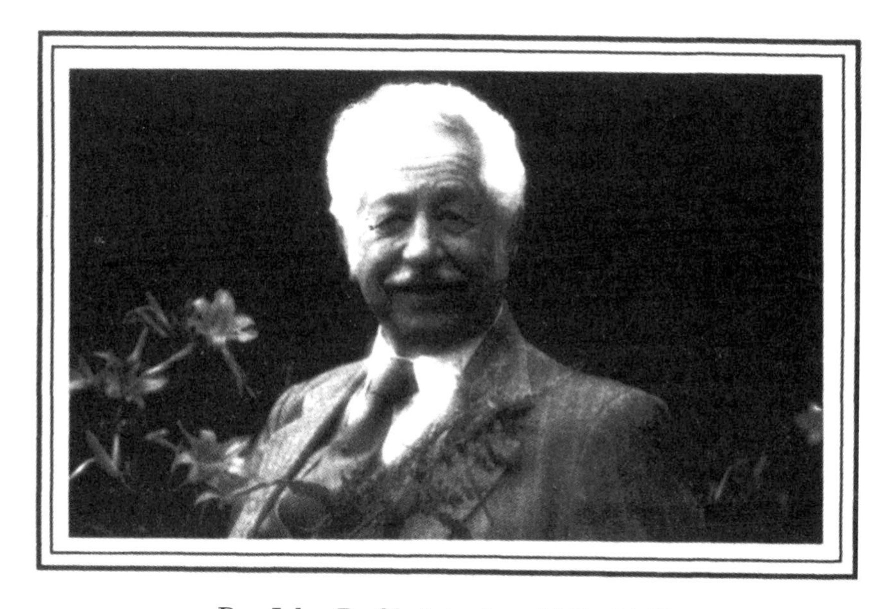

Dr. John R. Christopher, N.D., M.H.
November 25, 1909 — February 6, 1983

Dedicated in loving memory of Dr. John R. Christopher. A friend, who taught me by example that to truly live a life of purpose is to be in service of those who are sick or in need, or are less fortunate. To have respect for all life whether it be human, animal, plant or other forms. He has given me a deeper love and respect for our healing friends of the Plant Kingdom. It is my hope that we may all strive to live a life dedicated to becoming true human beings—a life full of purpose!

> *"...and the fruit thereof shall be for meat and leaf thereof for medicine."*
>
> —*Ezekiel* 47:12

Disclaimer

This book is a reference work and is not intended to treat, diagnose, or prescribe. All the herbs in combinations or singly have been used traditionally and historically and are passed on to the reader for educational purposes. The author and/or publisher assume no responsibility for any adverse effects or consequences resulting from the use of any remedies, procedures, or preparations included in this Herbal First Aid Book. This information is presented only for its educational value and should not replace the services of a competent, holistic physician when his services are required.

While taking these herbs, singly or in combinations, a warning is given not to use any stimulants including drugs, alcohol, coffee or sugar.

Acknowledgements

A special thanks to my wife Janae, for her unconditional love and support, and to my loving sons and daughters, Aubrey, Jared, Deserae, Ariel, Jadon, Destiny, Jordan and Jonathan. Thanks for sharing your life with me.

Foreword

Kurt and I sat down together recently, swapping herb stories, discussing case histories, and exchanging remedies. In the course of our reunion, and after much discussion, we decided that a usable book on herbal first aid was greatly needed.

Because of time restraints, I bowed out of the project and encouraged Kurt to write the book. After reviewing the book I can say that he's put together a wonderful guide to not only first aid but health care in general.

One of the great attributes of this work is in its simplicity. Natural healing is not a complicated subject, and neither is first aid.

My next praise for this book can be taken from the hippocratic oath, "First, do no harm." Herbs are the safest most effective tool available for health care. Unlike drugs, which have a myriad of side effects that can and do cause harm, herbs can be used with confidence and you will do no harm.

Many people are aware of the wonderful tonic effect of herbs that, when taken in small quantities over a long period of time, miraculously correct old chronic conditions; but as Kurt brings out in *Herbs to the Rescue,* herbs can work just as fast and even more effective than patented, synthetic drugs in dealing with acute emergencies.

At the risk of sounding trite, let me say, study this book, use this book, and please "don't leave home without it."

David W. Christopher, MH
Director, The School of Natural Healing

Introduction

During the past few years many things have happened to me and my family to change our way of thinking and looking at life. In response to what has taken place in my life, I have been motivated to write this book, "Herbs to the Rescue: An Herbal First Aid Handbook."

After many years of study and examining what I call "visionary visions" by various spiritual people of all walks of religion and race, I have discovered they are all saying the same thing. Unless people change and start using the Golden Rule as a standard, we are not going to survive as a human family into the 21st Century. Or in other words, people need to seek more of a spiritual fulfillment rather than instant gratification through materialism or the living spirit within us is going to die.

These "visionary visions" are telling us that if we, as a people, don't change our directional outlook, there is going to be much trouble for the people of the earth. We are beginning to see a lot of it already in the forms of earthquakes, famine, plagues unknown to mankind before now, bloodshed, and destruction of the earth. But if we don't change, it's going to get worse, much worse.

Still, we do have the power to change. One person can make a difference, and does. It could be said that when you help one person you are helping the whole world, so don't despair thinking there is no hope. "As long as there's one light shining there is hope for the world."

So let our hearts be tuned to our Creator, our fellowman, and our Mother Earth, and work towards healing each other and our planet. We must put human beings and living things first before the acquisition of material items. The "visionary visions" say if we do these things that we can offset what awaits us.

We know that "When the animals and plants die, man will soon follow." –Tom Brown, Jr. I wrote this book as a "what if." What if there was no electricity? What if food distribution is shut down? What if there is a national disaster? What if you had to survive in the woods? What if you were attacked by an enemy and had to flee? (An old enemy that has lost everything is the most feared enemy.) Think these things through and visualize how you would deal with them.

This book is only a beginning. Search out other books on first aid, survival, and self-sufficiency so you can be prepared for the times of "what if." And work to bring about a change in people's hearts and attitude as I have dedicated my life to doing. But I am also taking steps to be prepared for "what if..."

Working for a Better World where truth doesn't need to be defended, truth stands on its own. It is my prayer that the creator guards your paths in the near future.

—Kurt King, M.H.

Table of Contents

PART I

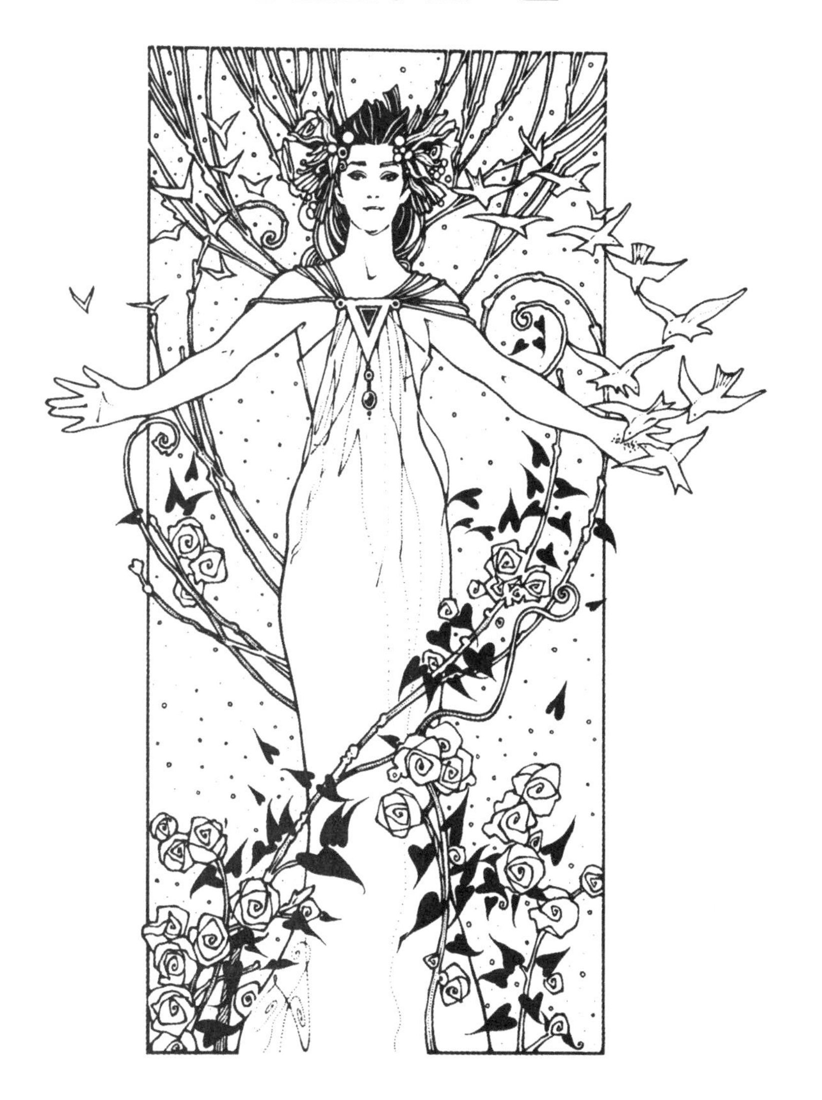

One person, one idea, one thought can turn the flock of society away from the destructive path of modern times. It is not a question as to whether we make a difference, for we all make a difference, each of us in our own way. It is the difference we make that is important.

—Stalking Wolf (The Quest)

PART ONE

Herbal First Aid

First Things First

1. Stay calm and **think first** before you act.
2. Check if person is breathing and if there is a heartbeat. (Pulse check on wrist or neck arteries. Visually notice chest action for breathing.) If person is not breathing or pulse cannot be found, administer emergency CPR immediately.
3. Check for severe bleeding (hemorrhage).
4. The next priority is to examine for shock (Shock is a serious condition of acute circulatory collapse, usually brought on by severe blood loss or trauma). Then examine for head injuries, fractures, lacerations and dislocations.
5. Begin treating person accordingly using a good "bed-side manner," calming and reassuring the person to help prevent shock or hysteria.
6. Find adequate shelter for the injured person, out of the harsh elements. Keep person warm, calm and reassured that all is going well.

Herbal Doses

All recommended doses are for adults. Use ½ dose for teenagers (13-16), ¼ dose for children (6-12), ⅛ dose for babies (2-6), and 1/16 dose for infants under 2 years.

NOTE: Where multiple herbs are listed **In the Woods** (herbs commonly found in nature), one or all can be used separately or in conjunction for teas, poultices or fomentations. (Use equal parts in combination.)

Conditions and Herbal Remedies

(In alphabetical order)

ABSCESSES

Black Ointment
Applied directly to the abscess to draw out toxins, then apply **X-Ceptic Tincture.** Apply **Complete Tissue & Bone (C.T.B) Ointment** to area of abscess until skin returns to normal.

Lobelia Tincture
Dose: 3-5 drops 2 times a day, internally.

Yarrow Tincture
Dose: 15-20 drops, 3 times a day, internally.

IN THE WOODS

Use fresh Yarrow or Plantain as a poultice over abscess. Drink Yarrow or Plantain tea 2-5 cups a day.

ACNE

Nettle Tincture
Dose: 10-15 drops 4 times a day, internally.

IN THE WOODS

Drink Dandelion Root tea, also Plantain tea 2-4 cups a day. Wash skin with Nettle Leaf tea 2-3 times a day.

ALLERGIES

Virutean (Super Garlic Immune Formula)
Dose: 10-12 drops 3 times a day, internally. Relieves hay-fever, respiratory allergies and swollen membranes. Also helps cleanse the body (skin rashes).

X-Ceptic Tincture
Dose: 10 drops on infected areas. Then apply **Complete Tissue and Bone Ointment** to skin until it returns to normal.

Nettle Tincture
Dose: 10-15 drops 3 times a day, internally.

IN THE WOODS
Drink Nettle and Mullein teas 2-4 cups a day.

ANEMIA

Nettle Tincture
Dose: 15-20 drops 4 times a day, internally.

IN THE WOODS
Drink Dandelion Root, Yellow Dock, Nettle teas, 3-4 cups a day. Also drink Yarrow tea to help build and cleanse the blood.

ANXIETY

Ear & Nerve Tincture
Dose: 15-20 drops 4 times a day.

IN THE WOODS
Drink Horsetail and/or Catnip tea 3-4 cups a day.

APPENDIX (Complaints)

(Mild Attack)
Raspberry Leaf tea
Dose: 2-4 cups a day until irritation stops.
(Severe Attack)
Catnip tea enema or lukewarm water to move waste material out. Apply **Lobelia Tincture** and hot Castor Oil packs over appendix area, elevate feet. Then apply hot and cold

packs of water over area until attack is over.
Drink 2-4 cups **Lower Bowel** made into tea.

IN THE WOODS

Catnip tea enema or luke-warm water to move waste material out. (On an empty stomach) Drink Nettle tea 2 to 3 cups, elevate feet and apply cold water packs over the appendix area. Apply poultice of Plantain and Yarrow over appendix area. If fever, use Yarrow tea 2-3 cups a day. (**Special Note:** An enema bag should be included in your survival kit for emergencies such as appendicitis.)

APPETITE, Loss of

Yarrow Tincture
Dose: 10-15 drops in a cup of hot water 2 times a day.

IN THE WOODS

Sage, Yarrow tea 2 cups a day. Any bitter herb will help with digestion which will then help with appetite.

ARTHRITIS

Horsetail Tincture
Dose: 10-15 drops 4 times a day.

Nettle Tincture
Dose: 10-15 drops 3 times a day.
Use Cayenne Heat Ointment topically for relief of muscular inflammation and joint aches.

IN THE WOODS

Yarrow, Nettle, Horsetail singly or in equal combinations, 2-4 cups a day.

ASTHMA

Nettle Tincture
Dose: 10-12 drops 2 times a day.

Lobelia Tincture
Dose: 3-5 drops 2 times a day.

Garlic Oil
Dose: 10-12 drops 2 times a day.
(Severe Attack)
Lobelia Tincture
Dose: 1 tsp.-1 tbsp. to induce vomiting.

IN THE WOODS

Drink 3-4 cups Mullein tea a day. Also drink 2-3 cups Nettle tea a day.

ATHLETE'S FOOT

(Jock Itch, Foot Fungus, etc.)
Super Garlic Immune Tincture over affected area. Apply **Complete Tissue and Bone Ointment** on area, or if affected area is extra moist, sprinkle **Ginger Root Powder** after applying **Super Garlic Immune Tincture.**
(Ringworm)
Apply **Sen-Sei Balm.** If pus develops, use **Echinacea Tincture** and **Garlic Oil** topically. For fingernails and toenails, use **Nettle Tincture** topically and 10-12 drops 3 times a day, internally. Additionally use **Black Walnut Tincture** topically.

IN THE WOODS

Drink 2-3 cups of Nettle and Yarrow tea. Also soak feet in warm tea.

BACK PAIN

Yarrow Tincture
Dose: 10-12 drops in hot cup of water 3 times a day. Apply **Cayenne Heat Ointment** over painful area. (If pain in lower right or left sides, or both persists, possible kidney complaint. Use **Horsetail Tincture** 10-15 drops 3 times a day.)

IN THE WOODS

Yarrow tea, Horsetail tea, 2-3 cups a day.

BEE STINGS (Insect bites, spider bites)

X-Ceptic Tincture topically and **Black Ointment** to draw out poisons, then **Complete Tissue and Bone Ointment.** If it gets sore and swollen, apply **Echinacea Tincture** topically and take internally.
Dose: 10-15 drops 4 times a day.

IN THE WOODS

Use a Plantain poultice over bite to draw out poisons. Drink Plantain tea, 2-4 cups; Yarrow tea 2-4 cups as hot as you can drink it. (For more detailed information on **Insect Bites (Poisonous),** see Appendix.)

BLADDER

Horsetail Tincture
Dose: 10-15 drops 3 times a day.
Nettle Tincture
Dose: 10-15 drops 2 times a day. **Lobelia Tincture** applied topically over painful area.

IN THE WOODS

Horsetail, Nettle tea, combination of equal parts 4 cups a day. Bed straw can also be used.

BLEEDING

Apply pressure directly on the wound to help stop blood flow. Internally, use **Cayenne Tincture** 10-12 drops in conjunction with **Horsetail Tincture** 10-15 drops every few minutes until blood flow stops. Typically, use **Cayenne powder** directly on wound.

IN THE WOODS

Shepherd's Purse, Yarrow or Horsetail poultice applied directly to wound. Also use any or all above herbs for tea to drink until bleeding stops. If infection develops, apply Plantain poultice. (For more information on **Bleeding (Severe),** see Appendix.)

BLISTERS

Use freshly-picked Plantain or Mullein leaves in your shoes to prevent foot blisters. If blisters develop, apply Plantain poultice. Use **X-Ceptic Tincture** to prevent infection and **Complete Tissue and Bone Ointment** to help heal.

IN THE WOODS
Plantain, Horsetail poultice

BLOOD PRESSURE (High or low)

Cayenne Tincture
Dose: 10-15 drops 2 times a day.
Shepherd's Purse Tincture
Dose: 10-20 drops 2 times a day.
Use Lobelia Tincture to lower blood pressure. Dose: 3-5 drops 2 times a day.

IN THE WOODS
Mistletoe, Shepherd's Purse tea 2-3 cups a day.
(Caution: Do not take Mistletoe if pregnant!)

BLOOD PURIFICATION

Echinacea Tincture
Dose: 10-12 drops 2 times a day.
Yarrow Tincture
Dose: 10-12 drops 2 times a day.
Nettle Tincture
Dose: 10-12 drops 2 times a day.

IN THE WOODS
Yarrow, Nettle, Plantain, Dandelion, Red Clover as tea 2-4 cups a day.

BLOODY NOSE

Put pressure on both sides of nose with cold compress. If it doesn't stop within 5 minutes, moisten a piece of cotton or gauze with water and dip it into Cayenne powder and stuff it into nose.

Internally, take **Cayenne Tincture**
Dose: 10-15 drops every 5-10 minutes until bleeding stops. (With a child, Cayenne may be too discomforting) use

Horsetail Tincture or Shepherd's Purse Tincture
Dose: 10-15 drops every 5-10 minutes.

IN THE WOODS

Use same pressure with cold compress. Drink Horsetail tea, Shepherd's Purse tea, Yarrow tea until bleeding stops.

BOILS

Nettle Tincture·, internally.
Dose: 15-20 drops 3 times a day.

Yarrow Tincture·
Dose: 10-12 drops 2 times a day.

Black Ointment topically.
Dose: Drink plenty of water and cleanse bowels.

IN THE WOODS

Drink Nettle, Yarrow tea 2-4 cups a day. Apply Yarrow or Plantain Poultice to affected area.

BREASTS

(Sore, Swollen, Infected, Cracked Nipples)
Hot Shepherd's Purse compresses over breast. Marshmallow Root or Leaf tea or Tincture to increase or enrich milk, also Alfalfa, Horsetail and Nettle.

Yarrow Tincture
Dose: 10-15 drops, 3 times a day. **Complete Tissue and Bone Ointment.** Apply Complete Tissue and Bone Ointment to affected breast. Sage tea for drying up milk when mother is ready to quit nursing.

IN THE WOODS

Hot Shepherd's Purse or Comfrey compresses for sore or swollen breasts. Marshmallow Root tea to increase milk. For sore nipples, expose breasts to sunshine. Apply Yarrow tea compresses.

BREATHING (Stopped)

Make sure air passage isn't blocked. (See detailed instructions on Heimlich Maneuver in Appendix) Administer Artificial Respiration. (See detailed instructions on **Breathing (Artificial Respiration)** in Appendix.)

BROKEN BONES (Simple fractures)

Horsetail Tincture
Dose: 15-20 drops 4-5 times a day, internally. Apply **Complete Tissue and Bone Ointment** over affected area. Put 2 splints on either side and wrap with gauze. Internally, **Super Garlic Immune Tincture**
Dose: 10-12 drops 3 times a day. (See physician if bone needs to be set).

IN THE WOODS
Set bone and splint, wrap with gauze. Drink Horsetail, Nettle, Alfalfa 2-3 cups a day to help knit bones.

BRONCHIAL DISORDERS

Ginger
Dose: Fomentation over chest area.

Lobelia Tincture
Dose: 2-3 drops 2-3 times a day.

Nettle Tincture
Dose: 10-12 drops 3 times a day.
(Bad Attacks)

Lobelia Tincture
Dose: 1 tsp.-1 tbsp. to help open up breathing passages, steam vapor using **Sen-Sei Balm.** Put small amount into a pan of boiling water. Cover head with towel and breathe in vapor.

IN THE WOODS
Drink Mullein, Nettle, Plantain tea, 3-4 cups a day. Burn Sage or Mullein and breathe in smoke to open up lungs.

BRUISES AND CONTUSIONS

Cayenne Heat Ointment
Dose: At night, dust area with **Ginger Powder** or **Slippery Elm Powder** to prevent itching or irritation. Then apply **Complete Tissue and Bone Ointment.**

IN THE WOODS

Plantain poultice over affected area. Drink Horsetail, Yarrow, Nettle tea, 2-3 cups a day.

BURNS

Grease
Remove all grease from burn with soap and water. Submerge burned area in cold water, or burns that cannot be submerged in water cover with wet, cold towels, changing them frequently. Use **Complete Tissue and Bone Ointment** or **Dr. Christopher's Burn Ointment** (See instructions for **Burn Ointment** below). Use **X-Ceptic Tincture** on burn 10-12 drops 3 times a day.

Chemical
Flush the burned area many times with tepid water for as long as 15-20 minutes. Treat herbally the same way as a grease burn.

Minor
Submerge the burned area immediately in cold water or apply cold, wet towels. Then follow the same instructions as with grease burns.

IN THE WOODS

Use Comfrey, Plantain, or Horsetail as a poultice. Also drink Horsetail and Comfrey tea, 3-4 cups a day.

Major
Treat person for shock (See Appendix for **Shock**). Cut around all clothing that has adhered to the skin (do not try to pull it loose). Apply Olive Oil or Vitamin E Oil to help with healing and to prevent pulling when bandages are changed. Then apply **Complete Tissue and Bone Ointment** and **Dr. Christopher's Burn Ointment** until completely healed. Use **Echinacea Tincture,** internally.

Dose: 25-30 drops 5-6 times a day.

Horsetail Tincture
Dose: 30-35 drops 2-3 times a day.
Take **X-Ceptic Tincture** and **Super Garlic Immune Tincture** to fight off infection.
Dose: 15-20 drops each 3 times a day.

IN THE WOODS
Use Comfrey, Plantain, Marshmallow, Mullein, Yarrow as a combination for a poultice. Drink Horsetail, Yarrow, Mullein, Plantain teas, 8-10 cups or more a day.

Dr. Christopher's Burn Ointment is made by mixing equal parts Honey, Comfrey Root Powder and Wheat Germ Oil. Mix together well and apply in a thick layer to burned area. Put on a dressing of gauze and tape it. Change bandages at least every four hours or as needed. Do this until the burn is healed. (This formula doesn't keep long, so make it fresh each day.)

CIRCULATION (Poor, cold hands & feet)

Nettle Tincture
Dose: 10-15 drops 3 times a day.
If you need something stronger, use **Cayenne Tincture**
Dose: 10-12 drops 2-3 times a day.

IN THE WOODS
Drink Nettle, Shepherd's Purse tea 2-4 cups 3 times a day.

COLDS/FLU

Super Garlic Immune Tincture
Dose: 10-15 drops 3 times a day.

X-Ceptic Tincture
Dose: 10-15 drops 2 times a day. Gargle with **Ginger Tea** and soak in hot **Ginger** bath. (**Cayenne Tincture** or **Powder** will also help.)

IN THE WOODS
Drink Nettle, Horsetail, Yarrow tea, 3-4 cups a day.

COLIC

Kid-e-Col
Dose: As needed

Ginger tea,
Dose: 1 cup a day. For small infants, use Catnip tea, **Catnip & Fennel Tincture** or **Kid-e-Col.**

Slippery Elm Gruel
Dose: As needed. (For adult use) Add water to Slippery Elm Powder to make paste. Then add more water for gruel-like consistency.)

IN THE WOODS
Drink Catnip, Horsemint tea.

CONSTIPATION

Nettle Tincture
Dose: 12-15 drops 1 hour before breakfast.

Lower Bowel
Dose: 2-3 tsp. a day or drink **Lower Bowel** tea, 2-3 cups a day. Eat more greens, vegetables, fruits and whole grains, less meat. Drink ¾ to one gallon of water a day. Take long walks to move bowels.

IN THE WOODS
Nettle tea, 1 hour before breakfast. Yarrow tea, 2-3 cups a day as hot as you can drink it. Also chickweed tea, 2-3 cups a day.

COUGHING

Plantain Tincture
Dose: 10-15 drops 3 times a day.

Lobelia Tincture
Dose: 3-5 drops 3 times a day. Gargle with tea made from **Herbal Tooth Powder, X-Ceptic Tincture** Dose: 10-12 drops 3 times a day.

IN THE WOODS
Plantain tea, 3-4 cups a day, Marshmallow tea, 2-3 cups a day.

CRAMPS

Menstrual:
Female Reproductive Formula
Dose: 10-15 drops 3 times a day.

Yarrow Tincture
Dose: 10-12 drops 2 times a day.

Ginger
Dose: 2 cups a day as a tea

Muscle:
Horsetail Tincture
Dose: 10-15 drops 4 times a day.

Nettle Tincture
Dose: 10-15 drops 3 times a day. Apply **Herbal Heating Balm** to affected area.

Stomach:
Ginger
Dose: 2 cups a day as a tea.

Nettle Tincture
Dose: 10-15 drops 3 times a day.

IN THE WOODS

Menstrual:
Yarrow, Horsetail tea, 2-3 cups a day.
Shepherd's Purse, 2 cups a day.

Muscle:
Horsetail, Nettle tea, 3-4 cups a day.

Stomach:
Catnip tea, 2-3 cups a day.

CUTS

If bleeding, apply pressure. Use **Cayenne Powder** to stop bleeding. Make sure cut is clean of all foreign matter. Apply **X-Ceptic Tincture** and then **Complete Tissue and Bone Ointment** bandage with butterfly bandages if wound is deep.

IN THE WOODS

Use Horsetail, Yarrow, Shepherd's Purse, Plantain poultice to stop bleeding and help heal. Also drink as tea, 2-3 cups a day.

DEPRESSION

Ear & Nerve Tincture
Dose: 10-15 drops 4 times a day to feed the nerves.

Horsetail Tincture (To add calcium to the system.)
Dose: 10-15 drops 3 times a day.

Mind Trac
Dose: 2 capsules 3 times a day

Kid-e-Trac
Dose: 10-15 drops 3 times a day

IN THE WOODS

Drink Horsetail tea, 2-4 cups a day. Also Nettle, Plantain, Catnip or Dandelion can be used. St. John's wort tea can also be used.

DIAPER RASH

Slippery Elm Powder or **Healing Clay Powder** over area, then apply **Plantain Ointment.** Expose area to sunlight. Mother should take internally, if nursing baby.

Echinacea Tincture
Dose: 10-12 drops 2 times a day. Also apply **Complete Tissue and Bone Ointment** to help heal skin.

IN THE WOODS

Use Plantain fomentation over area. (Also can use Plantain or Mullein leaves next to skin.) Mother should drink Horsetail and Nettle tea, 2-3 cups a day, if nursing.

DIARRHEA

Let the body do its work first. If the person becomes weak or dehydrated, stop the cleansing with **Lower Bowel** tea, 2 cups a day.

Yarrow Tincture
Dose: 10-15 drops 3 times a day. Chamomile tea, 2-3 cups a day. If diarrhea continues, use **Slippery Elm** gruel.

IN THE WOODS
Drink Yarrow, Catnip tea, 2-3 cups a day. Inner barks of Aspen, Larch, Birch, Oak made into tea will help stop diarrhea.

DROPSEY (Edema)

Nettle Tincture
Dose: 10-15 drops 3 times a day.

Horsetail Tincture
Dose: 10-15 drops 3 times a day.

IN THE WOODS
Drink Horsetail, Nettle tea, 4-6 cups a day.

EAR (Complaints)

Garlic Oil
Dose: 4-5 drops in ear, then place piece of clean cotton or wool in ear opening.

(Ears Ringing)

Ear & Nerve Tincture
Dose: 4-5 drops in each ear, then add Garlic Oil. Also will help with equilibrium problems, hearing loss, nerve damage.

IN THE WOODS
Hot Mullein leaf fomentation. Yarrow poultice over ear area.

ECZEMA

Black Ointment Applied on area at night.

Complete Tissue and Bone Ointment during the day.

Nettle Tincture
Dose: 15-20 drops a day, internally. Also apply **Garlic Oil** on infected area.

IN THE WOODS
Drink Nettle tea, 2-4 cups a day, Horsetail tea, 1-2 cups a day. Horsetail, Yarrow, Plantain can be used topically as a poultice.

EXHAUSTION (Fatigue)

Nettle Tincture
Dose: 15-20 drops 4 times a day, helps increase iron if anemic.

Cayenne Tincture
Dose: 10-12 drops 2 times a day.

IN THE WOODS
Drink Nettle tea, 2-3 cups a day. Also Alfalfa, Dandelion, Mullein tea will help increase energy.

EYE PROBLEMS

Herbal Eyebright Combination made into a tea, strain and wash out eye with it. Drink 1-2 cups of **Eyebright** tea a day. Helps sore, tired, infected eyes, poor vision.

IN THE WOODS
Yarrow fomentation over eyes at night. Drink Yarrow tea, 2-3 cups a day.

FEMALE DISORDERS

Female Reproductive Formula
Dose: 10-15 drops 3 times a day.

Yarrow Tincture
Dose: 10-12 drops 3 times a day.

Red Raspberry Leaf Tea
Dose: 2-3 cups a day

IN THE WOODS
Drink Yarrow tea, 2-3 cups a day. Also, for vaginal infection, douche with lukewarm Yarrow tea. For excessive bleeding, drink plenty of Yarrow, Horsetail, Shepherd's Purse tea.

FEVER

Echinacea Tincture
Dose: 10-15 drops 6 times a day.

Yarrow Tincture
Dose: 10-15 drops 4 times a day.

For infants: **Echinacea Tincture**
Dose: 8-10 drops into 4-6 oz. water in bottle.
Soak in hot **Ginger** bath. **Slippery Elm** tea is good for young and old in all cases of fever. Also cool water enemas with **Lower Bowel** 1-2 cups, to remove all poisons from the system. For extreme fevers, use an emetic (cause vomiting); **Lobelia Tincture,** 1-3 tsp. until it produces vomiting.
In all fevers use **Yarrow Tincture**
Dose: 10-15 drops 3 times a day or Yarrow tea, 4-6 cups a day. Elderflower and Peppermint tea is excellent for helping

with fevers. (For cold sheet treatment, see Dr. Christopher's Cold Sheet Treatment Book.)

IN THE WOODS

Drink one or more of the following until fever breaks: Yarrow, Nettle, Sage, Chamomile, Elderflowers, Raspberry, leaf tea. Also the inner bark of Birch, Larch, Aspen can be made into a tea and drank. (Make sure bowels are clean, with cool enemas.)

FLATULENCE (Gas, stomach and bowels)

Ginger tea
Dose: 1-2 cups a day.

Lower Bowel tea
Dose: 1-2 cups a day.

Yarrow Tincture
Dose: 10-15 drops once a day.

IN THE WOODS

Drink Catnip, Yarrow, Horsemint tea, 2-3 cups a day.

FROSTBITE

(Mild)
Apply **Cayenne Heat Ointment** over area and wrap. **Cayenne Tincture**, internally.
Dose: 10-20 drops 4-6 times a day.

(Extreme)
If the person's skin is white or grayish with no pain, just tingling or numbness, do not massage the frostbitten area, but bring the person to a place out of the elements. Then warm the area by immersing it in hot water (104°F-108°F).

IN THE WOODS

Apply Mistletoe poultice over affected area. Drink Nettle tea, 4-6 cups a day. (For more detailed information on **Frostbite,** see Appendix.)

FUNGUS

(Under Finger and The Nails)

Nettle Tincture
Dose: 10-15 drops 3 times a day, internally. Externally, soak nails in Nettle tea or apply **Nettle Tincture.**

(Ringworm)
Apply **Sen-Sei Balm** over affected area. Also **Black Ointment** and **Garlic Oil** over affected area.

IN THE WOODS
Drink Nettle, Plantain tea, 2-3 cups a day. Use fomentation of the herbs over affected area and also rinse hair with tea if scalp is affected.

GALL BLADDER (Complaints)

Lower Bowel tea
Dose: 2-3 cups a day.

Nettle Tincture
Dose: 10-15 drops 3 times a day.

IN THE WOODS
Drink Nettle tea, 3-4 cups a day, 1 cup a half-hour before breakfast. Hot fomentation over affected area of Nettle, Plantain, Mullein, Dandelion, Oregon Grape Root.

GANGRENE

Burns from fire or acid, frostbite that is not properly cared for, and any wound that becomes stagnant with waste matter in the system can turn into gangrene.
Mortification or death to the soft tissues sets in with the failure of the local blood supply. The inflammation or drying tissues are bluish or black in color, and yellow or black spotting with dry gangrene, when the circulation is very poor. People with poor circulation or who have blood that is not clean, run a greater risk of getting gangrene.

Lower Bowel tea.
Dose: 2-4 cups a day.

Cayenne Tincture
Dose: 10-15 drops 4-6 times a day. Nettle Tincture Dose: 10-15 drops, 4-6 times a day to increase circulation. Soak the affected area with Marshmallow root tea, as hot as the person can tolerate. Use a poultice or fomentation of Oregon Grape Root, Marshmallow, Plantain, Nettle, Horsetail, Oak or Poplar bark. Keep person calm, warm, and well-nourished.

IN THE WOODS
Cleanse the colon with Catnip tea enema. Drink 1 cup Nettle tea first thing in the morning. Also drink Yarrow, Nettle, Plantain, Shepherd's Purse tea, 4-8 cups a day (Helps circulation). Follow same instructions above for soaking and poultice/fomentation.

GLANDS (Swollen)

Ecbinacea Tincture
Dose: 10-15 drops 3 times a day.

Lobelia Tincture
Dose: 1-3 drops 2 times a day. Typically, rub **Lobelia Tincture** into skin, where gland is swollen, then apply **Plantain Ointment.**

IN THE WOODS
Drink Yarrow, Oregon Grape, Plantain tea. Make poultice of Plantain, Mullein leaves.

GUMS (Bleeding, loose teeth, inflammation)

X-Ceptic Tincture
Dose: 10-12 drops 3 times a day.

Horsetail Tincture
Dose: 10-15 drops 3 times a day. Apply **Herbal Tooth Powder** to gums and gargle with tea.

IN THE WOODS
Drink Horsetail tea, 2-3 cups a day. If infected, drink Nettle, Yarrow, Plantain tea, 2-3 cups a day. Also put the bruised herbs (above) on affected gums. Chewing on inner bark of Oak, Larch, Poplar and Birch will also help.

HEADACHES

Drink **Lower Bowel** tea, 2-3 cups a day. (Constipation is a major cause for headaches. Cleanse colon with lukewarm enema.) Apply **Sen-Sei Balm** on temples. Drink Catnip, Chamomile tea if stress headache.

IN THE WOODS

Drink Yarrow tea, 2-3 cups a day. Chew on Willow or Poplar Bark (or small twigs). You can also drink Nettle, Catnip, Mullein tea for relief of headaches.

HEART (Heart attack, palpitation)

Cayenne Tincture
Dose: 1 dropper under tongue. Massage **Cayenne Heat Ointment** on arm.

(To strengthen heart) **Horsetail Tincture**
Dose: 10-15 drops 3 times a day.

Nettle Tincture
Dose: 10-12 drops 3 times a day.

IN THE WOODS

(To strengthen) Drink Nettle, Horsetail, Alfalfa, Red Clover tea, 3-4 cups a day.

HEART FAILURE

Check for pulse. If no pulse can be found, administer CPR (cardio-pulmonary resuscitation). This life-saving procedure requires training and practice. Check your area to see where CPR classes are available. (Usually taught at hospitals or YMCA. For a brief outline of **CPR** techniques, see Appendix under CPR.)

HEAT STROKE

If the person's body temperature is 105° or higher, pour cold water over entire body, head to feet. Give cool drinks and wrap in cold, wet sheets of cloth until body is cooled down. (For more detailed information on **Heatstroke,** see Appendix.)

HEMORRHAGE (Heavy Bleeding)

For detailed information on how to treat **Hemorrhage (Heavy Bleeding),** see Appendix.

HEMORRHOIDS

Yarrow Tincture
Dose: 10-12 drops 2-3 times a day.

Horsetail Tincture
Dose: 10-15 drops 4 times a day. Apply **Complete Tissue and Bone Ointment** topically over affected area.

IN THE WOODS
Drink Yarrow, Horsetail, Plantain tea, 2-4 cups a day. Apply fomentation of above herbs over area. Inner barks of Oak, Larch, Poplar, Birch as a tea and a lukewarm enema will help, also as a fomentation.

HERNIA

Complete Tissue and Bone Ointment
Dose: Applied at night over affected area. Use **Healing Clay** poultice mixed with **Horsetail Tincture** also over area.

Internally, **Horsetail Tincture**
Dose: 10-20 drops 3 times a day.

IN THE WOODS
Drink Horsetail tea 4-6 cups a day. Also Horsetail, Shepherd's Purse fomentations over area.

HERPES

Echinacea Tincture
Dose: 10-15 drops, 3 times a day. Apply **X-Ceptic Tincture** on fluid-filled blisters. Then apply **Complete Tissue and Bone Ointment** until after scabbing stage is over. Can also apply Healing Clay sprinkled over area before applying the **Complete Tissue and Bone Ointment.**

IN THE WOODS
Drink Yarrow tea, 3-4 cups a day, also Horsetail tea, 2-3 cups a day.

HYPOTHERMIA

Cayenne Tincture
Dose: 1 dropper under tongue.

Nettle Tincture
Dose: 1 dropper under tongue. In all cases of hypothermia, the body core temperature must be warmed as quickly and safely as possible (Direct body contact, warm baths, warm drinks, etc. are all recommended methods). Do not warm extremities before body core is warmed first! Keep victim in adequate shelter, away from wind and elements. Make sure they are dry and comfortable. (For more detailed information, see **Hypothermia** in Appendix.)

HYSTERIA

Ear & Nerve Tincture
Dose: 10-15 drops 3 times a day.

Horsetail Tincture
Dose: 10-15 drops 3 times a day.

IN THE WOODS
Drink Horsetail, Catnip, Yarrow tea, 4-6 cups a day

INDIGESTION

Nettle Tincture
Dose: 10-12 drops 3 times a day.

Ginger tea
Dose: 1-2 cups a day.

IN THE WOODS
Drink Nettle, Catnip, Dandelion, Alfalfa tea, 3-4 cups a day.

INFECTIONS

X-Ceptic Tincture, internally
Dose: 10-15 drops 3 times a day. Use **X-Ceptic Tincture** topically over area, sprinkle with powdered **Ginger** and apply **Black Ointment** to area.
Use **Garlic Oil** internally.
Dose: 10-15 drops 3 times a day, and externally over infected area.

IN THE WOODS
Drink Plantain, Yarrow, Oregon Grape tea, 3-4 cups a day. Make poultice from above herbs and apply to area.

INSECT BITES

Echinacea Tincture
Dose: 15-20 drops 3 times a day. **Apply Black Ointment** or **Plantain Ointment** over bite that has been cleaned.

IN THE WOODS
Apply Plantain poultice over bite area. Drink Plantain, Yarrow, Horsetail tea, 3-4 cups a day. (For more detailed information on **Insect Bites (Poisonous)** see Appendix.)

INSOMNIA

Ear & Nerve Tincture
Dose: 10-12 drops 4 times a day.

Horsetail Tincture
Dose: 10-15 drops 3 times a day. Take your shoes off and walk on grass or bare earth.

IN THE WOODS
Drink Horsetail, Catnip tea, 3-4 cups a day. Walk barefoot on bare earth.

JAUNDICE

Yarrow Tincture
Dose: 10-15 drops 3 times a day. Lower Bowel tea. Dose: 2-3 cups a day. Expose person to direct sunlight. (Especially good for infants.)

IN THE WOODS
Drink Yarrow, Plantain, Nettle, Dandelion, Oregon Grape Root tea, 3-6 cups a day.

KIDNEYS (Complaints)

Super Garlic Immune Tincture
Dose: 10-12 drops 3 times a day.

Horsetail Tincture
Dose: 10-15 drops 3 times a day.

Nettle Tincture
Dose: 10-15 drops 3 times a day.

IN THE WOODS
Drink Marshmallow, Nettle, Horsetail, Dandelion tea, 3-4 cups a day.

LIVER (Complaints)

Lower Bowel tea.
Dose: 2-3 cups a day.

Yarrow Tincture
Dose: 10-12 drops 3 times a day.

Plantain Tincture
Dose: 10-12 drops 3 times a day.

IN THE WOODS
Drink Yarrow, Plantain, Nettle, Dandelion, Oregon Grape Root tea, 3-4 cups a day.

MASTITIS

Echinacea Tincture
Dose: 20-30 drops 3 times a day. If fever, **Yarrow Tincture.**
Dose: 20-30 drops 3 times a day. Use hot fomentation of Mullein and Shepherd's Purse over affected breast.

IN THE WOODS
Drink Plantain, Yarrow tea, 3-6 cups a day. Use Marshmallow, Yarrow, Shepherd's Purse, Plantain for poultices.

MUSCLES (Pulled, strained)

Cayenne Heat Ointment over affected area. If torn, apply **Complete Tissue and Bone Ointment** on area.

Internally, **Horsetail Tincture**
Dose: 10-15 drops 3 times a day. **Shepherd's Purse Tincture** applied to area.

IN THE WOODS
Drink Horsetail, Nettle tea, 3-4 cups a day. Apply Shepherd's Purse, Horsetail, Plantain fomentations over affected area.

NERVOUS DISORDERS

Ear & Nerve Tincture
Dose: 15-20 drops, 4 times a day.

Horsetail Tincture
Dose: 10-15 drops, 3 times a day.

IN THE WOODS
Drink Horsetail, Catnip, Nettle tea, 2-3 cups a day.

POISONING (By mouth)

First, identify the poison if possible. If it is a strong corrosive poison or petroleum product, **do not induce vomiting.** Give plenty of fresh water or milk to drink. If it is not a strong corrosive poison or petroleum product, **induce vomiting** by giving them 1-3 tsp. of Lobelia Tincture, Or by gagging with finger in back of throat. Then give them plenty of fresh water to drink.

Use **Black Cohosh Tincture.**
Dose: ½ to 1 dropper to neutralize poison. Then use **Echinacea Tincture**
Dose: ½ to 1 dropper. Keep the person calm and warm, sitting up in a comfortable position. If **unconscious,** or **convulsing,** do not administer anything by mouth, but **seek medical attention, immediately.**

IN THE WOODS

Same procedure as above. (Where applicable. For detailed instructions on **Poisoning from Snakes or Insects,** see Appendix.)

POISON IVY, OAK & SUMAC

Wash the area with soap and water and make sure affected clothing is removed. Apply **Black Ointment** to affected area, and cover with gauze (This ointment is messy and stains clothing).

Internally, use **Echinacea Tincture**
Dose: 10-20 drops, 3 times a day.

Black Cohosh Tincture
Dose: 10-20 drops, 3 times a day. Drink Catnip tea, 2-3 cups a day.

If fever, use **Yarrow Tincture**
Dose: 10-20 drops, 4 times a day. (Caution: If pregnant, do not take Black Cohosh Tincture)

IN THE WOODS

Use Plantain, Mullein poultice or fomentation over affected area. Drink Plantain, Nettle, Yarrow, Catnip tea, 3-4 cups a day.

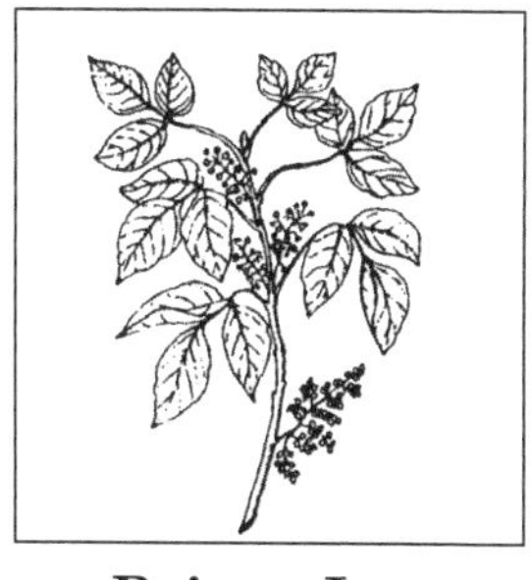

Poison Ivy

Throughout U.S. (except California). The leaves are shiny and grow in groups of three, turning red/ yellow at fall time.

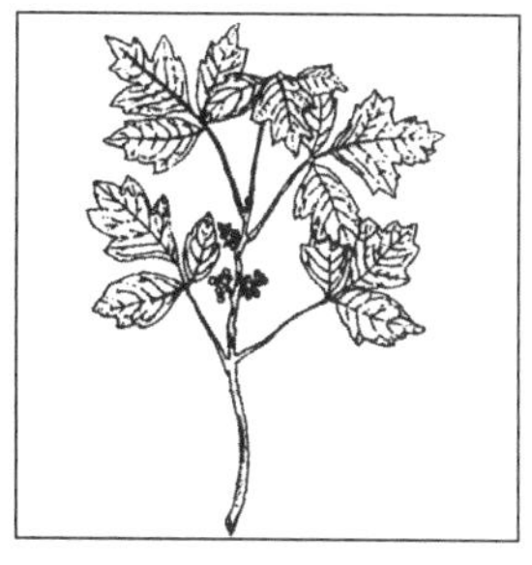

Poison Oak

Western variety grows in California, and it is found in adjacent states. The more common variety grows in different parts of U.S. Shrub / clusters of hairy, yellowish berries. The underside of leaves are covered with hair.

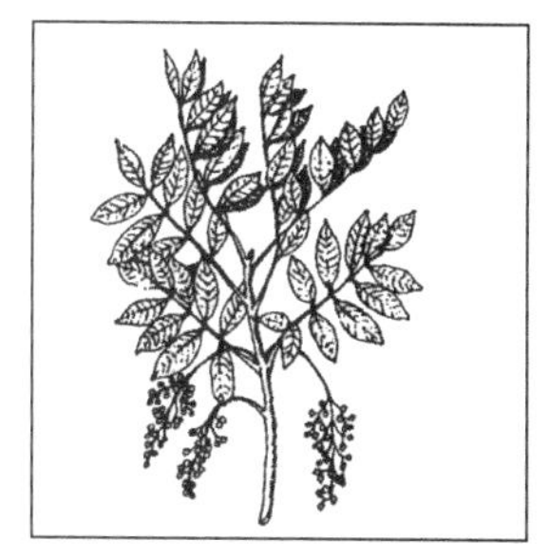

Poison Sumac

Shrub or small tree – 5-25 ft, found in eastern U.S. Cream-colored berries in loose clusters turn red in fall. Individual leaf stalk has 7-13 leaflets with smooth edges.

PNEUMONIA

Plantain Tincture
Dose: 10-12 drops into a hot cup of water 3-4 cups a day.

Super Garlic Immune Tincture
Dose: 5-10 drops 3 times a day.

Cayenne Tincture
Dose: 5-10 drops, 3 times a day.

Garlic Oil
Dose: 10-15 drops, 3 times a day.

IN THE WOODS

Drink Plantain tea as hot as you can drink it, 2-3 cups a day. Drink Yarrow tea, 2-3 cups a day.

PROSTATE (Complaints)

Lower Bowel tea.
Dose: 2-3 cups a day.

Garlic Oil
Dose: 10-15 drops 3 times a day.

Yarrow Tincture
Dose: 10-12 drops 3 times a day.

Slippery Elm Powder made into a gruel adding water.
Dose: 1-2 tsp. 2-3 times a day. lukewarm enema to clean bowels.

IN THE WOODS
Drink Yarrow, Nettle, Horsetail tea, 3-4 cups a day. If swollen, Mullien, Plantain fomentation over area.

RADIATION POISONING

Yellow Dock & Bugleweed Combination Capsules or Tincture.
Dose: 4-6 capsules or 10-12 drops 3 times a day.

American Ginseng Tincture.
Dose: 15-20 drops 3 times a day. Bathe in 2 lbs. Epsom Salt water for 1 hour, then 2 lbs. soda water for 1 hour.

Healing Clay
Dose: 1 tsp. in a glass of water, let sit overnight, then drink it. Eat foods with Iodine or Selenium in them.

IN THE WOODS
Drink Yellow Dock, Nettle, Yarrow tea, 4-6 cups a day.

RASHES AND SKIN ERUPTIONS

Plantain Tincture
Dose: 10-15 drops 3 times a day.

Yarrow Tincture
Dose: 10-15 drops 3 times a day.

Echinacea Tincture
Dose: 10-12 drops 3 times a day. **Apply Plantain**

Ointment over affected area.

IN THE WOODS

Drink Plantain, Yarrow, Chickweed, Dandelion, Mullein tea, 3-4 cups a day. Wash affected area with Plantain tea.

SHOCK

Administer 1 dropper of **Cayenne Tincture** under tongue, followed by 1 dropper of **Nettle Tincture.** Make sure person is warm and dry and lying flat on back with feet elevated.

IN THE WOODS

If person can swallow, administer Nettle, Shepherd's Purse tea, as hot as you can drink it. Use same procedure as above. (For more information on Shock, see Appendix.)

SNAKEBITES (Poisonous)

For detailed information on **Snakebites (Poisonous)** and how to treat, see Appendix.)

SPLINTERS (Pieces of metal, glass or wood)

Remove splinter with sterile tweezers. Apply **X-Ceptic Tincture** over wound. If imbedded, apply **Black Ointment** mixed with **Healing Clay** to draw out splinter.

IN THE WOODS

Remove splinter. Apply Plantain poultice over wound. If imbedded, warm Pine Sap applied to wound will draw out splinter.

SPRAINS

Cayenne Tincture
Dose: 5-10 drops 2 times a day.

Horsetail Tincture
Dose: 10-12 drops 3 times a day. Externally apply **Cayenne Heat Ointment** to affected area for relief.

IN THE WOODS
Drink Nettle, Yarrow, Horsetail tea, 3-4 cups a day. Use Mullein, Horsetail poultice over area. Use Comfrey leaf poultice if available.

STOMACH (Complaints)

Drink **Ginger** tea 2-3 cups a day.

Nettle Tincture
Dose: 10-12 drops 3 times a day.

IN THE WOODS
Drink Nettle, Yarrow, Catnip tea, 3-4 cups a day. (Also see Constipation, Cramps, Flatulence, Indigestion.)

SUNBURN

Complete Tissue and Bone Ointment over area every 4-6 hours.

Horsetail Tincture, internally.
Dose: 10-12 drops 3 times daily.

IN THE WOODS
Wash area with Nettle, Horsetail tea. If blistered, apply Plantain poultice. Drink Horsetail, Nettle tea, 3-4 cups a day.

TETANUS (Lockjaw)

At onset of tetanus, **Lobelia Tincture.**
Dose: 15-20 drops, 2-3 times to induce vomiting, followed by Cayenne Tincture Dose: 5-10 drops. Ear & Nerve Tincture Dose: 15 drops, 2 times a day.

Lobelia Tincture

Dose: 3-5 drops 2 times a day.

Echinacea Tincture
Dose: 10-12 drops 3 times a day.

Super Garlic Immune Tincture
Dose: 10-12 drops 3 times a day.

IN THE WOODS
To induce vomiting, use 1 or 2 fingers applied to the back of throat until stomach is emptied. Then drink Nettle tea, 2-3 cups a day followed by Horsetail tea, 4-6 cups a day. Yarrow tea, 2-3 cups a day as hot as you can drink it. Apply Plantain poultice over wound if there is a puncture of the skin.

THROAT (Infection, sore)

Gargle with **Herbal Tooth Powder** made into a tea.

Garlic Oil
Dose: 10-15 drops 3 times a day.

X-Ceptic Tincture
Dose: 10-12 drops 3 times a day. Apply **Sen-Sei Balm** on outside surface of throat for relief.

IN THE WOODS
Make strong tea of Plantain leaves, gargle and drink 2-3 cups a day.

TICKS

Remove tick and apply **X-Ceptic Tincture** and **Garlic Oil.** Also apply **Plantain Ointment** over area. (For more detailed instructions on **Tick (Removal),** see Appendix.)

ULCERS

Cayenne Tincture
Dose: 10-15 drops 2 times a day and **Slippery Elm** powder made into a gruel by adding water, for stomach ulcers.

Horsetail Tincture
Dose: 15-20 drops 3 times a day. Horsetail, Plantain poultice for skin ulcers.

IN THE WOODS

Drink Horsetail, Plantain, Shepherd's Purse tea, 2-4 cups a day. Horsetail, Plantain poultice for skin ulcers.

UTERUS (Disorders, prolapse)

(Uterine Hemorrhages)

Horsetail Tincture
Dose: 10-15 drops 3 times a day.

Shepherd's Purse Tincture
Dose: 10-15 drops 3 times a day.

Yarrow Tincture
Dose: 15-20 drops 3 times a day to normalize periods.

(Prolapsed Uterus)
Empty colon with lukewarm enema. Massage abdomen area with **Shepherd's Purse Tincture** starting with the vagina and working upward.

IN THE WOODS

Drink Horsetail, Yarrow, Shepherd's Purse tea, 3-4 cups a day. Apply Shepherd's Purse fomentation over uterine area.

VIRUS INFECTIONS

Super Garlic Immune Tincture
Dose: 10-15 drops 3 times a day, or more if needed.

Echinacea Tincture
Dose: 10-12 drops 3 times a day. When assisting people with contagious diseases, it's a good idea to put some Ginger Root or **Ginger Powder** between your gum and lip to ward off disease.

IN THE WOODS

Drink Plantain, Yarrow, Nettle, Oregon Grape Root tea, 3-4 cups a day.

VOMITING

To stop: Lobelia Tincture
Dose: 2-6 drops.

Ginger tea
Dose: 1-2 cups a day.

To induce:

Lobelia Tincture
Dose: 1 tsp. to 1 tbsp. to rid stomach of toxins. After vomiting, use **Nettle Tincture**
Dose: 15-20 drops to restimulate circulation.

IN THE WOODS

To stop:
Catnip, Nettle, Horsemint tea, 2-3 cups a day.

To induce:
Drink 5-6 cups of lukewarm water. Vomiting should come on. If not, press finger to back of throat. Continue until stomach is empty. Note: Vomiting should be induced when it is necessary to empty the stomach or cleanse the stomach of poisons or toxins in cases of fevers, nausea, food poisoning, being bitten by rabid dogs, poisonous snakes, or poisonous insects, Also, if tetanus is setting in, to get all toxins out of the body, an enema should also be used.

WORMS

Garlic Oil
Dose: 15-20 drops, 3 times a day.

Healing Clay
Dose: 1 tsp. in a glass of water, let sit overnight, then drink it.

IN THE WOODS
Drink Tansy, Nettle, Horehound tea 3-6 cups a day.

WOUNDS

Use **Cayenne Powder** or **Tincture** to stop bleeding, then apply **X-Ceptic Tincture** or **Echinacea Tincture** over wound. Cover with **Complete Tissue and Bone**

Ointment and bandage until wound heals. (Change bandages regularly.)

IN THE WOODS

Use Horsetail, Yarrow, Shepherd's Purse poultice to stop bleeding. Wash wound with Yarrow tea. Bandage and drink Horsetail, Nettle, Yarrow tea, 3-4 cups a day. (For more detailed information on **Wounds,** see Appendix.)

PART II

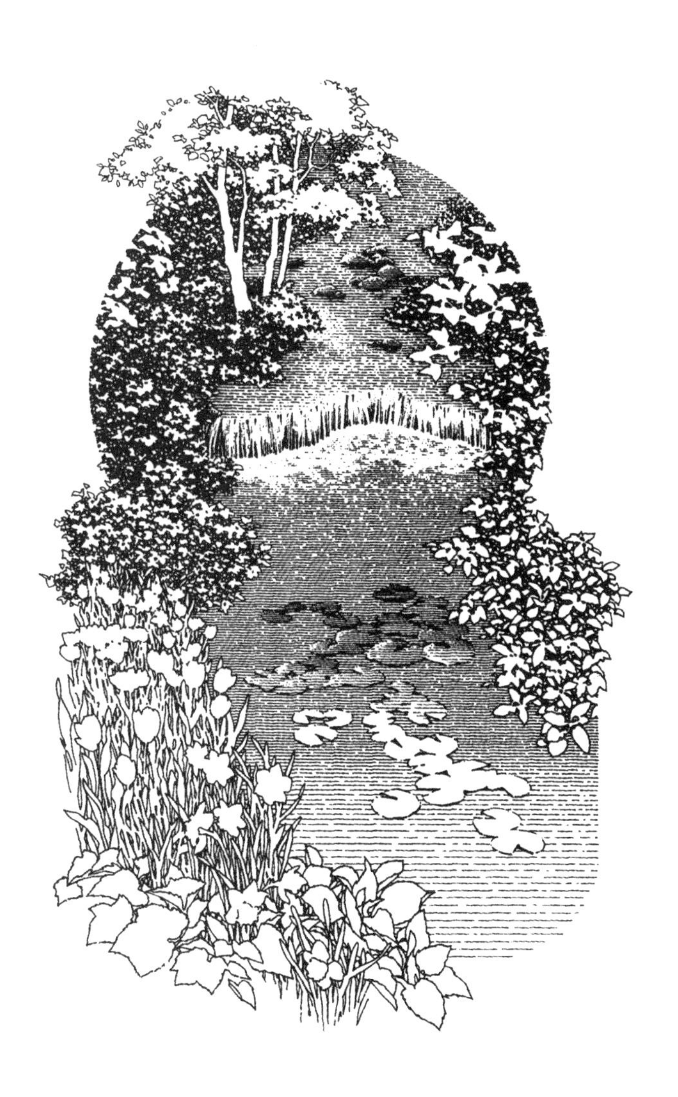

"There is a wonderful science in nature, in trees, herbs, roots, and flowers, which man has never yet fathomed. In nature, God has provided a remedy for every disease that might affect us."

—Jethro Kloss, Back to Eden

PART TWO
Out in the Field and Forest
(Thirteen Easily Available Herbs for Survival)

As I contemplate the perhaps **difficult times ahead,** the following **13 herbs** would be the ones I would choose for my family to become familiar with. I share these with you, the reader, in the hopes that they may be a **blessing** to you as they have been for my family and myself.

As an herbalist, I have studied hundreds of herbs, but very few have I gotten to know in a very personal way. As I have gotten to know these **13 herbs** for survival, my awe for the **"Spirit** that moves within all things" has deepened with greater love and **respect.** I view these herbs as **Healing Friends** from the **Creator.**

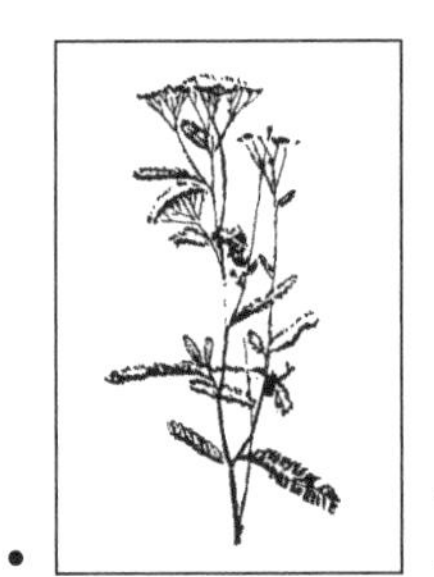

1. Yarrow *(Achillea millefolium)*

I begin first with one of the most **sacred** and **powerful** of all herbs-**Yarrow.** It was said around 120 years ago by a visionary, holy man that when **troubled times** came, if you had this **sacred** herb you would be able to ward off **any type of plague** or **fever.**

Yarrow is a **powerful healer** and **purifier.** Its fragrance seems to reach deep down inside you pulling forth the impurities within. Its distinct aroma and appearance makes it easily identifiable in the field. Filagree leaves and clusters of tiny white flowers are its distinct characteristics when foraging for **Yarrow** in the fields.

Yarrow has been extremely beneficial in many types of disorders. It does wonders for the **female reproductive organs, regulating menstruation** in younger women and helping older women through difficulties in **menopause.** It has been my experience that **every woman** with any female complaint could benefit by drinking one cup of **Yarrow tea** a day.

Yarrow also helps with **abdominal disorders, nose bleeding, migraine headaches, blood cleansing** and **renewal, bone marrow disorders, bleeding** of the **lungs, bleeding hemorrhoids, stomach bleeding, indigestion** and **heartburn, colds/flu, gas, liver disorders, constipation, lack of appetite, fevers, skin infection, boils, pimples,** etc. You may now begin to appreciate why the old herbalists called **Yarrow "a cure for all ills."**

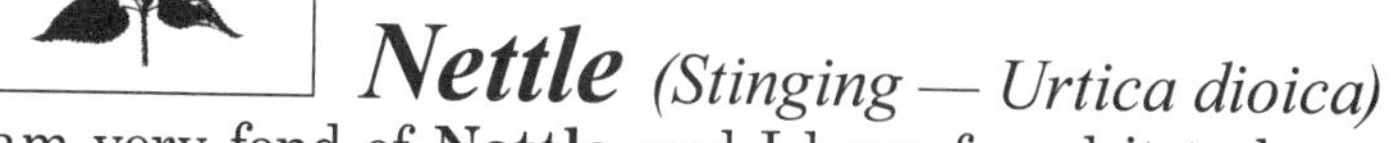

2. Nettle *(Stinging — Urtica dioica)*

I am very fond of **Nettle** and I have found it to be one of the most **valuable medicinal herbs** in the field. Many people are somewhat leery of using **Nettle** because of its "stinging" reputation, but if handled with care (gloved-hands suggested) it can be one of the most **vibrant** plants there is. Its jagged-edged and square stem marks its distinctions.

Being a person who loves the outdoors and exerts high amounts of energy on long hikes in the mountains, I call **stinging Nettle** my **natural energizer.** It acts like a **mild Cayenne** in **stimulating circulation** and reviving a weary body. Not only is it great for **fatigue** and **exhaustion,** but it keeps my circulation at its best as I never have **cold hands** or feet. Nettle is great for the blood due to its **high iron content** and its high levels of **vitamins A and C** and **protein. Nettle** is also good for **liver, gall bladder** and **spleen disorders,**

headaches, dropsy, anemia, blood disorders, colds/flu, allergies, vascular constrictions, faulty circulation, eczema, blood cleansing and **building,** stimulates the **bowels** and **urinary tract,** helps the **pancreas.** Also can be used as a hairwash to **stimulate hair growth.**

I regularly drink 1 part **Nettle,** 1 part **Horsetail,** and 2 parts **Chamomile** made into a tea to maintain health and well-being.

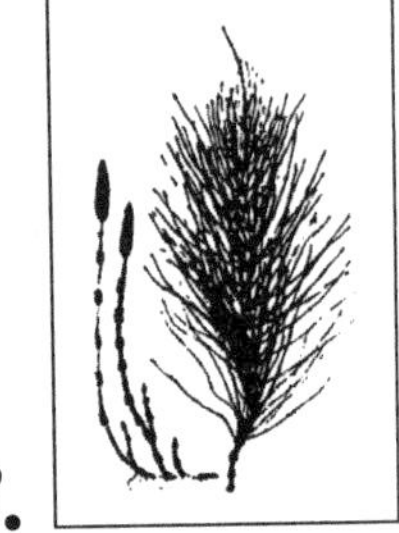

3. Horsetail *(Equisetum aroease)*

I esteem **Horsetail** as the most valuable herb for **building calcium** in the body and **preventing arthritis** and **rheumatism**-like pains. Its appearance is two-fold. In its first year it appears like a bristly horse's tail which is how I prefer to use it as it is more tender and has more medicinal qualities. The tall reed-like, matured **Horsetail** can also be used, but with less value as the chlorophyll is decreased and also some of the vitamins and minerals.

Horsetail has always been one of my favorites for **kidney** and **bladder** troubles. I am reminded of a story of a man in his late 70's who **couldn't urinate** and was so swollen up with an **accumulation of water** that he couldn't walk without help or even see his ankles from so much swelling. He went to the hospital and got no results. By way of his son, he received some **Horsetail** to make into a tea. He cussed and said he wasn't going to take "any blasted weed," but eventually his son convinced him to try it. The following morning the older man, still cantankerous and cussing, said he didn't sleep well at all that night as he had to keep getting up and going to the bathroom. Then he realized he could see his ankles and walk without aid which really made him a **believer** of **Horsetail.**

Horsetail is most **helpful** when all other **diuretics fail.** I have used it with amazing results for all **pain** caused by **rheumatism, arthritis** and **gout.** I have also used it for **leg**

cramps and **hemorrhaging** in **childbirth** with excellent results. **Horsetail** is also good for **ulcerated legs, dropsy, itching rashes, herpes, hemorrhoids, visual defects, nervousness, nose bleeds, bedwetting, depression, bursitis, bleeding gums, tonsillitis,** disorders of the **lungs, uterus** and **stomach,** and **chronic bronchitis.** I feel very thankful to the **Creator** for giving us such a wonderful herb as **Horsetail.**

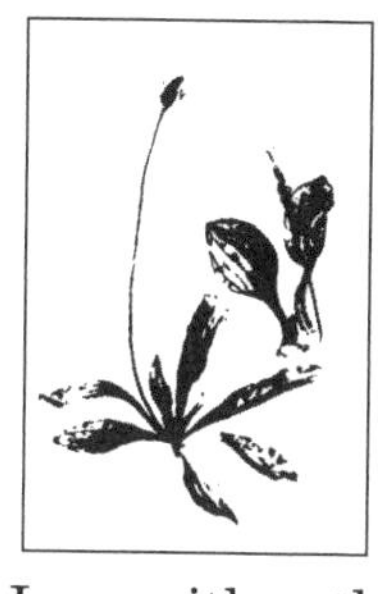

4. *Plantain* *(Platago lanceolata, Plantago major)*

I use either the **broad leaf** or the **narrow leaf Plantain** in the same medicinal way. Both are distinct in that the veins in the leaves run parallel from stem to tip. There is a legend in India that tells of how the **mongoose,** after being **bitten** by the **deadly cobra,** goes off into the field or forest to find its **antidote—Plantain.**

Another old herbal saying tells that when "a **toad** is **bitten** by a **spider,** it hurries to find **Plantain** for help."

What a marvelous teacher is nature and its wildlife, if we would only **look, listen** and **learn.** And what a marvelous **blood cleanser** is **Plantain,** especially when it comes to **poisonous bites** and **stings.** (Although I have yet to try it on a cobra bite!) It is Nature's remedy for **dog bites, cuts, scratches, wounds, blisters, bee** and **wasp stings, open oozing sores,** and all **skin maladies.** It is also great for the **lungs, bronchitis, bronchial asthma,** and phlegm in the **lungs.** Eating the seeds and leaves can strengthen weak children and adults. It also acts as an **internal insecticide,** possibly making the skin odorless and tasteless to insects.

So next time you walk out on the lawn, notice the humble **Plantain** plant and offer a little prayer for such a helpful friend.

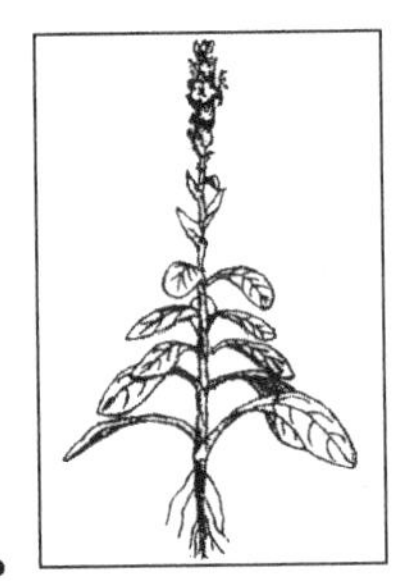

5. *Mullein* *(Verbascum thapsus)*

What a **proud** and **majestic herb** is **Mullein.** Near our log cabin in the woods we have a lot of **Mullein** growing, and in late summer the stalks of **Mullein** look like myriads of people standing in the forest. But there is one extremely large and majestic plant which we call **"The Grandfather"** plant which is the guardian of them all. We honor this plant by never using its leaves or flowers, but allowing it to grow unmolested.

For winter survival the dried stalks make excellent tinder and will ignite easily. They are also excellent for making a bow-drill fire apparatus, and the leaves make excellent padding for shoes or bedding. **Mullein** seeds have been used to catch fish in ponds when thrown in, as they are narcotic and cause a temporary stupor in fish.

Mullein also has many wonderful medicinal uses. Dried, the leaves can be smoked to ease **throat** and **lung congestions.** They can also be made into a tea for a similar effect. The flowers and leaves have been used for **bruises, frostbite, hemorrhoids, earaches, blisters, mastitis, stomach cramps, digestive system** disorders, **skin wash,** and are marvelous for easing and soothing **pain.**

Though stately and proud, the **Mullein plant** is also **soothing** and **calming.** The leaves are so soft and pliable that no herbal survivalist can resist plucking one or two on the way **"just in case of an emergency."**

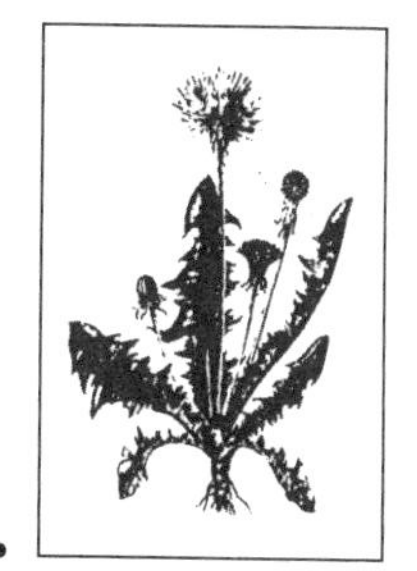

6. *Dandelion* *(Taraxacum officinale)*

Each year with the arrival of spring comes the arrival of one of the most **useful herbs known to man** – the **Dandelion.** And yet how many homeowners do everything in their power to rid themselves of this pesky "weed"? We try sprays and chemicals, spades and shovels, breaking our backs in order to create a perfectly manicured lawn. Yet in all our ignorance do we realize the value of the **Dandelion** as one of **Nature's greatest healing herbs?**

I was once sharing my beliefs and devotions concerning herbs with an older man who I would visit on occasion. He was in the hospital at the time suffering from **chronic inflammation** of the **liver** and **hepatitis.** I told him about **Dandelion** and what marvelous **healing** properties it had for the **liver.** He smiled and listened, but said he would rather trust in the doctors instead of some "noxious weed." Three days later he **died** of failure of the liver. I often think of this man when the **Dandelions** come out in the spring. He had **so much to live for,** but wouldn't **trust** in **Nature** to **heal him.** It saddens me to tears to think he could be alive right now if he would have only given herbs a chance.

Dandelion is a **good friend** to the **survivalist** and much needed for **suffering mankind.** It's a good tonic to be taken year-round as a tea. The **fresh stems** will bring quick relief to **chronic inflammation** of the **liver.** It helps relieve **stomach cramps, stimulates** the **liver** and **gall bladder,** it is a **blood purifier, diuretic,** helps chronic **skin disorders** such as **rashes, eczema** and **acne.** It helps the flow of **gastric juices** and added to salads makes a great health aid due to its high amounts of **Vitamin A.** It is also good for **poor eyesight,** and **night blindness.** People with chronic fatigue should try drinking **Nettle** and **Dandelion** tea 3-5 cups daily.

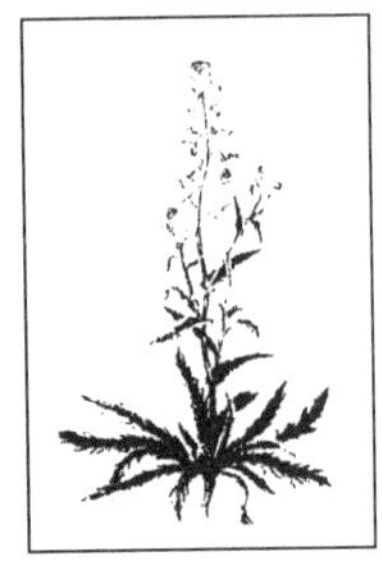

7. *Shepherd's Purse* *(Capsella bursa-pastoris)*

Shepherd's Purse, named for its unusual, heart-shaped seed pod, can be found almost anywhere. So when the situation arises where someone is **bleeding** from a **cut** or **wound** you can almost rest assured that **Shepherd's Purse** will be close by.

We have used it to stop **bleeding** during **childbirth** with much success. Also for **bleeding** of the **nose, stomach, intestines, uterus** and **hemorrhoids.** It also helps to regular excessive **menstrual flow,** and one lady I know used it as a douche for **fibroid tumors** of the **uterus.** The tea will also stimulate the bowels and kidneys. **Shepherd's Purse** is excellent for equalizing **blood pressure, high** and **low.**

For relief of an **earache,** crush the plant to a pulp. Put several drops into the ear canal and place some sterile cotton or paper over the ear opening. For **nose bleeds,** chew or crush up the plant to a moist pulp and insert into bleeding nostrils.

This herb is a must on camping trips or on a hike when accidents are bound to happen. Used internally and externally, bleeding should never be **life-threatening** if you're familiar with the properties of **Shepherd's Purse.**

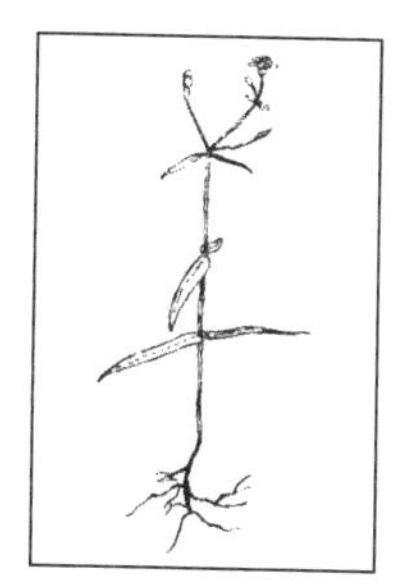

8. *Chickweed* *(Stellaria spp.)*

Chickweed is one of the most widely distributed plants in the world. It can be found in almost every lawn or garden and is characterized by its thin, winding vines with tiny white flowers.

We have used it for all kinds of skin disorders ranging from **rashes, abrasions** and **bruises** to **boils, blisters** and **burns.** It is also a remedy for **constipation** and helps to move the **bowels.** For **bronchitis** or **sinus headaches, Chickweed** will help without **drying** out the **nasal passages.**

9. *Elderberry* *(Sambucus canadensis)*

The **Elderberry** can be found throughout the United States and as far north as Canada. A beautiful, impressive shrub, its limbs seem to reach out to you along nearly every country road saying "**Partake** of my **healing virtues.**"

The first story I ever heard concerning **Elderberry** was told to me by **Dr. Christopher.** He told a story of a family in the early 1920's who had **tried everything** else to save their **feverish, dying infant.** Then they were told by a friend to use **Elderberry flowers** and **Peppermint** because not even in the last hours of life would this combination fail. They gave it a try and sure enough the baby **pulled through.**

I have used it on many occasions to alleviate fevers due to colds and flu. Wounds can also be helped by washing them with the tea.

Elderberry flowers are also good to cleanse the blood, for

headaches and **upset stomachs. (Warning:** The leaves and roots are poisonous. Unripe fruit can cause diarrhea and vomiting). Also, by mixing **Elderberry flower** tea with tallow, it can make a good drawing salve for **boils** and **splinters.**

The ripe berries can be lightly boiled and mashed and used for **burns.**

The blooming **Elderberry** bushes are a lovely sight to behold on long hikes and drives through the country. Who could ever guess that such loveliness would produce such a treasure trove of herbal delights.

10 . Mint *(Mentha spp.)*

What can compare to the **aromatic pleasures of** a cup of hot **Mint tea?** Both taste and aroma combine together to create a **spiritual uplift** and **calming** effect to the nerves. And have you ever watched a cat or kitten play in a patch of **Catnip**? It seems to energize them. **Peppermint, Spearmint, Horsemint** and **Catnip** have many different uses but all the members of the **Mint** family have similar characteristics. They can all be identified by their distinct aromatic smells and their jagged leaves and square stems.

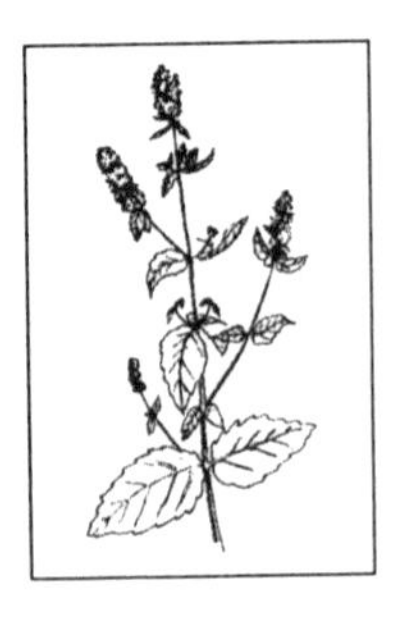

Catnip— Used for **soothing** the **nerves, digestion, colic,** enemas to pull out toxins, **fever, gas, stomach acid,** and to help **urination.**

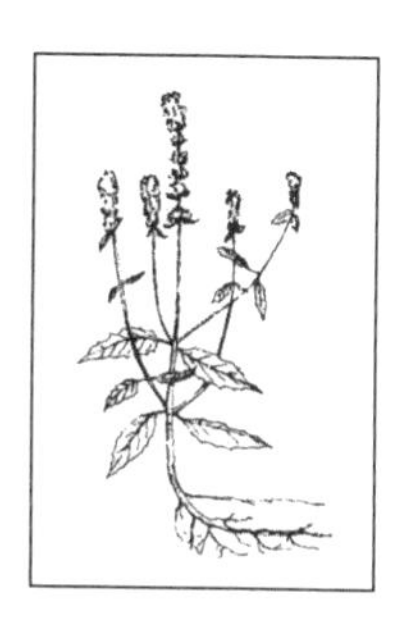

Peppermint— Remedy for **toothache, nausea, colic, gas, headache, insomnia, fevers** and **dysentery.** Makes a delicious tea.

Spearmint— Used for the same conditions as **Peppermint** but is especially good during **pregnancy** when **Peppermint** isn't tolerated.

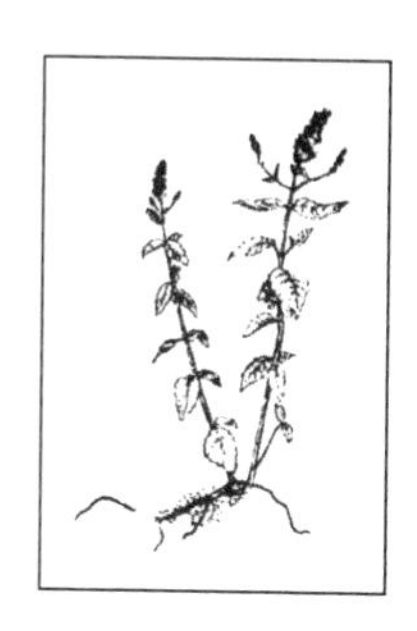

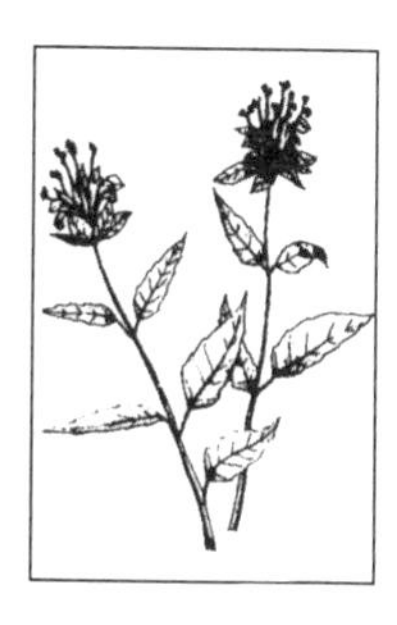

Horsemint— This "field" mint is easily available and is good for **colds, colic, gas,** and **diarrhea.** It is a delicious addition to any medicinal herb tea.

Pennyroyal— Used for **colds, flu, fever, jaundice, gas** and **epilepsy.** (Caution to pregnant women: The oil should never be used and the dosage should not exceed more than 1-2 cups of tea a day.)

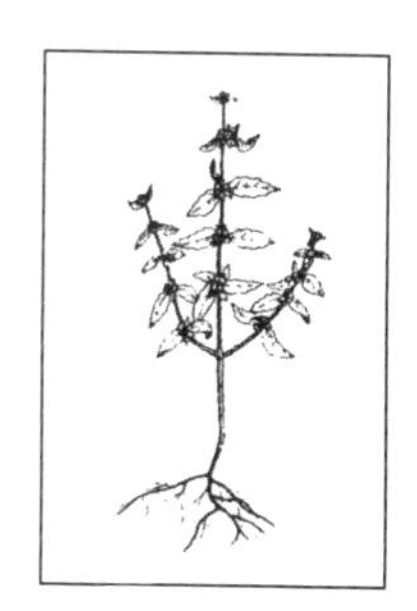

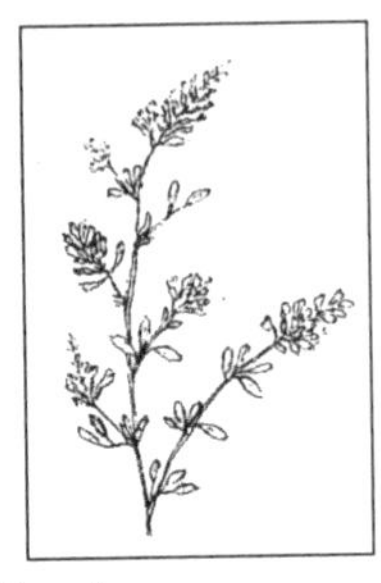

11. *Alfalfa* *(Medicago Sativa)*

Used as a crop for all livestock, we see how powerful and strong the horse and ox are, that it isn't surprising that **Alfalfa** is found to be high in **many vitamins** and **minerals.** This **"King of Herbs"** has been cultivated on over 27 million acres in the United States alone. It has been used by man for thousands of years for both food and medicine. In folk medicine, **Alfalfa** is acclaimed as a **"cure all"** for all **wasting diseases** and for **inflammations.** It is highly regarded as a **mild laxative** and aids in digestion due to a digestive enzyme (betaine).

Alfalfa has a deep tap root sometimes reaching down as far as 30 ft. It extracts many vitamins and minerals from the earth such as vito A, vito E, vito K, biotin, folic acid, pantothenic acid, zinc, selenium, magnesium, potassium, and silicon.

It's most popular use in American herbology is for **inflammation** due to **arthritis.** It is also used for **cleansing the blood, stimulating the appetite,** and as a **tonic** for all **wasting disorders.** Externally, it is used for **burns, cuts, bruises,** and to prevent scar tissue from forming. It has also been known to heal skin tissue damaged by **radiation.**

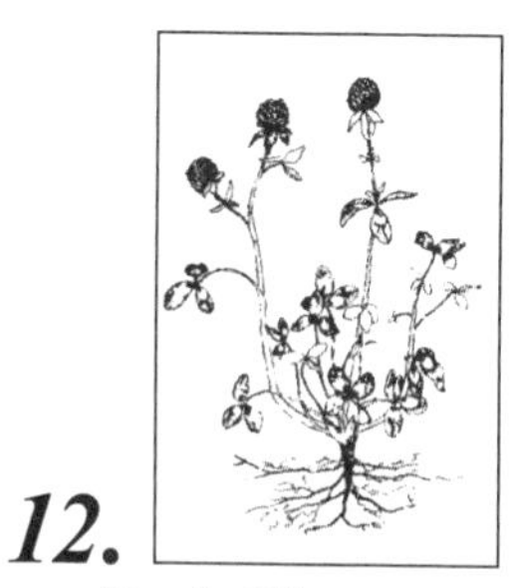

12. Red Clover *(Trifolium Pratense)*

Red Clover seems to be found everywhere in the United States. It is in the same noble family as alfalfa (Leguminosae or pea family).

Dr. Christopher, Chief Sundance, and Harry Hoxsey made this herb well-known in the U.S.A. All of these men, independent of each other, used this herb in their cancer formulas because of its effects on **purifying the blood.**

Red Clover is very high in **potassium, chromium, manganese, phosphorus, calcium, magnesium** and **niacin.** Because of its high amounts of **chromium** it protects the heart, and is essential in producing **glucose tolerance factor (G.T.F.)** which is necessary in the **production** and **utilization of insulin.**

Red Clover has traditionally been used to **clean the blood** and **expell any waste** in the system. It also helps **move mucous** out of the **lungs.**

Red Clover has a **calming effect** on the whole **nervous system** and is one of the **best herbs** we have to assist in **chronic illnesses** both in adults and children. Truly it is a **friend** to have and to hold.

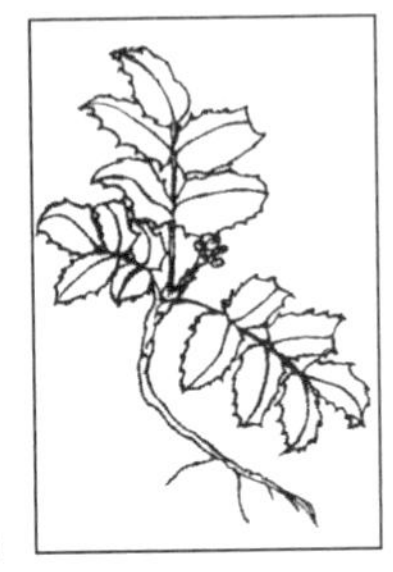

13. *Oregon Grape Root*

(Mahonia (Berberis) Repens)

Oregon Grape has been confused with so many other plants that I feel a brief description is in order.

The plant's leaves are rough, somewhat prickly around the edges, usually with seven to nine leaflets in pairs along a thin, tough stem. The blossoms are light yellow clusters, blooming in the spring; when ripe, the berries are dark blue. The evergreen leaves turn red in the fall, hence the Spanish name, **"Herb of the Blood."** This creeping ground cover plant seldom rises more than an inch or two above the ground. It can be found throughout the western U.S.

Because of the bitter alkaloid **berberine** in **Oregon Grape,** it works as an **antiseptic** and **antibacterial.** It is useful in **lowering fevers,** swollen and infected conditions, a **laxative** and **intestinal strengthener;** as an antibacterial skin wash for skin disorders; as a **liver stimulant,** for **gall-bladder** complaints, and a good **blood purifier.**

The flowers are good for a skin dressing to prevent infections. The berries can be made into a tea for **fevers, colds/flu;** and as a **laxative.**

Because of its many marvelous uses, **Oregon Grape** is one of the most beneficial medicinal plants in the western part of the U.S.

In conclusion, it is **my suggestion** that you get to **know** these **13 herbs intimately** and have them on **hand** either **dried** or in **tincture** form. You never know when you're going to **need them** and **your life** and your **family's lives** could depend on them.

PART III

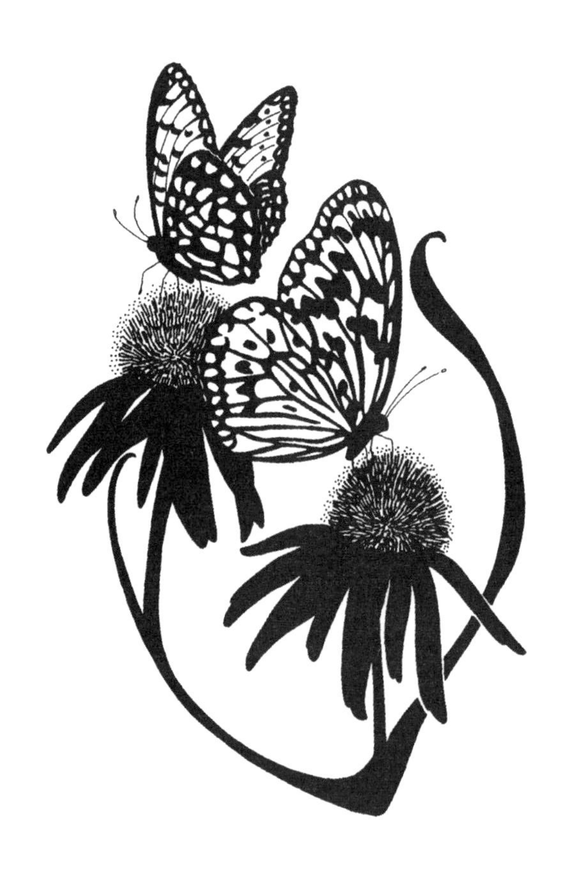

It is not dying that should be our fear, but man should fear having never lived at all.

—Marcus Aurelius

PART THREE

Healthful Reminders

* When faced with any illness, the best thing to do is to go on a mild food diet. For faster healing, whether it be a life-threatening illness or not, we have found you get better results (See Dr. Christopher's Three-Day Cleansing Program). This diet would include all natural, unrefined foods except dairy products, eggs, meat, and processed grain.

* **Attitude** — "As a man thinketh, so is he." **Attitude** is **everything** when it comes to survival. An archeologist by the name of Donald Grayson of the University of Washington did a study which showed that **women** are twice as likely as men to survive extreme cold and hunger. He based his research on the Donner Party, 19th century pioneers who resorted to cannibalism to survive the winter when trapped in the Sierra Nevada Mountains. One of the reasons was basic personality differences; (1) Women are more cooperative and less aggressive than men. (2) Women don't lose their tempers as easily as men. (3) Women have a greater percentage of fat that insulates them against the cold. (4) Women consume energy less quickly than men. (5) Women have a way of holding things together for longer periods of time. Grayson said that faced with the same type of famine and cold temperature conditions, Americans today would suffer a much worse fate than those of the Donner Party. "Most Americans are out of shape and flabby they're not as tough as the people in the Donner Party?" It's important that you not only develop **physical stamina,** but also a **positive mental attitude.** Practice thinking and visualizing yourself through any adverse situation. When lost in the woods,

most people would survive if they would just take the time to **sit down** and **think things through** in a positive light instead of acting out of blind panic.

As an herbalist and natural healer I have come to the conclusion over the years, that **your thoughts affect your health** more than anything else. When times of trouble come (and we all know they will) we should prepare ourselves by starting right now in becoming a more positive, happy human being. We must learn to take responsibility for our lives and happiness and then go out and serve those who are less fortunate than ourselves.

Childbirth — Emergency

Childbirth is a **natural process** so **never** try to hurry or force the birth. Make sure the area where the baby is to be born is as **clean** as possible and any instruments have been sterilized by boiling or immersing in rubbing alcohol. Also, wash hands thoroughly with soap (if possible).

During the birthing process, try to **remain calm** and **reassuring** to the mother.* Remember, she is the one doing most of the **work;** your job is that of an assistant. Most complications during delivery occur when nature is interfered with, so **never interfere** with the natural birthing process.

When the baby starts to move down the birth canal, have the mother lie down in a comfortable position on a soft, yet firm, surface (bedding or towels if available). As the head begins to emerge, assist the mother by **supporting** the **perineum** (the area between the vaginal opening and anus) with one hand to prevent the skin from tearing. With the other hand, support the baby's head as it emerges. **NEVER** pull on the baby's head in order to speed up the delivery, but wait for the contractions and mother's pushing action to facilitate the birth. As the head emerges, check to see if the **umbilical cord** is **wrapped** around the baby's neck. If it is, gently slip it over the baby's head. When completely delivered, the baby should be held with his **face down** or to the side to permit him to sneeze and cough out any mucus that may be in the nose or throat. If the baby is **blue** or **pale** and **not breathing,** gently administer **artificial respiration** by bending the **whole body** like a **hinge** so that the hips are brought towards the shoulders at the rate of once every five seconds. Mouth to mouth **resuscitation** is also recommended if the attendant is trained in this method as applied to infants.

If the umbilical cord is long enough, wrap the baby in a clean cloth to keep warm and give it to the mother to try and nurse (Nursing helps the uterus contract to help expel the afterbirth or placenta).

The afterbirth will follow the baby, usually in a few minutes, sometimes after many hours. If the woman isn't bleeding, don't do anything to hasten the delivery of the afterbirth. If there is some bleeding or cramping, you can gently massage the uterus which should bring on a contraction which will expel the afterbirth. **Never pull** on the **cord** to deliver the afterbirth.

After the afterbirth is expelled, make sure the mother isn't bleeding **excessively.** Normally the total amount of **blood loss should not exceed two cups.** The suckling of the baby at the breast will minimize blood loss. Manual compression of the uterus by holding it firmly together between two hands may be necessary in an emergency. Also Cayenne, Shepherd's Purse or Mistletoe can be administered in powdered or tincture form to stop a hemorrhage. Horsetail tea is also helpful.

The cord should not be dealt with until the placenta is delivered and the mother is out of danger, unless it is a short cord and won't allow for the mother to nurse. Make sure it has **stopped pulsating** and then tie a sterile string or piece of string around the umbilical cord about 3-4 inches from the baby. Tie a second string around the umbilical cord about an inch away from the first one. Cut the umbilical cord between the two ties with a sterile knife or scissors.

While the mother rests, the baby can be dressed or wrapped in a blanket to be kept warm. The natural grease should not be washed off the baby's body as it is a protective coating for the baby's skin. Of course, any blood or debris should be gently wiped away.

In The Woods

After conception and during pregnancy drink Raspberry leaf tea mixed with equal parts nettle and horsetail grass, 2-4 cups a day. Mint (spearmint, peppermint or chamomile) can be added for flavor and to help reduce nausea.

Nettle will help to build iron and Horsetail will help to build calcium both in the mother and baby.

Raspberry leaves help to nourish and strengthen all the female organs.

During delivery, make sure you have Shepherd's Purse tea and Horsetail Grass tea on hand to help with hemorrhaging. Also have Yarrow tea on hand in case of any infections.

* It is important that all those who are in attendance at a delivery be as quiet and peaceful as possible for the benefit of the mother and baby. If possible, the father should do the delivering as it creates a superior, natural bonding with mother and child. (I have personally assisted with all my children's deliveries and the last two my wife and I did ourselves. We found these to be the most rewarding of all the deliveries.)

The Colon: The Hub of the Wheel of Your Health

* **Signs of an Unclean Colon** — Gas, flatulence, foul breath, bad body odor, acne, digestive problems, infections of the kidney, prostate, bladder, liver and/or gall bladder, excess mucus in the head, lungs, and/or throat chronic sickness with all types of disorders.
* **To Cleanse the Colon** — Enemas help to clean out a bogged-down colon, help the colon rid itself of mucus and toxic matter, and help the colon to restore its peristalic action. When the colon is cleansed, many different disorders and ailments clear up on their own as the body can begin functioning the way it was designed to.

  When there is an illness of a chronic nature, one of the first steps to wellness is an enema. If there is a fever involved, use Catnip and/or Garlic.

  Use **Lower Bowel Formula.**

  Dose: 2-3 capsules 3 times a day.
* **Colon Maintenance** — To prevent the colon from becoming toxic and congested, it is recommended to keep on a mild food diet high in fruits, vegetables, and fiber. Use Psyllium as a natural laxative for occasional constipation.

Herbs Found in Book

Herbs *(Latin Names)*	**Parts Used**
Alfalfa *(Medicago sative)*	Leaves
Birch *(Betula fontinalis)*	Leaves, inner bark
Black Cohosh *(Cimicifuga racemosa)*	Roots
Catnip *(Nepeta cataria)*	Leaves & flower
Cayenne *(Capsicum annumn, Capsicum frutescens)*	Fruit
Chickweed *(Stellaria media)*	Whole plant
Comfrey *(Symphytum officinale)*	Leaves & roots
Dandelion *(Taroxacum officinale)*	Whole plant
Echinacea *(Ech. angustifola, E. purpurea)*	Whole plant
Elderberry *(Sambucus spp.)*	Flowers
Garlic *(Allium satiuum)*	Bulb
Ginger *(Zingiber officinale)*	Root
Horsemint *(Monarda fistulosa)*	Leaves & flowers
Horsetail *(Equisetum hyemale)*	Whole plant
Larch-Tamarac *(Larix Americana)*	Inner bark, needles
Lobelia *(Lobelia inflata)*	Seeds, leaves & flowers
Marshmallow *(Althaea officinalis)*	Root
Mistletoe *(Viscum album)*	Twigs & leaves
Mullein *(Verbascum thapsus)*	Leaves, seed & flowers
Nettle *(Stinging) (Urtica spp.)*	Leaves & flowers
Oak *(Quercus spp.)*	Inner bark
Oregon Grape Root *(Mahonia (Berberis) repens)*	Whole plant
Pennyroyal *(Hedeoma hispidum)*	Leaves & flowers
Peppermint *(Mentha piperita)*	Leaves & stems
Pine *(Pinus spp.)*	Inner bark, needles
Plantain *(Plantago major)*	Whole plant
Poplar, Quaking Aspen *(Populas spp.)*	Inner bark, leaves & buds
Shepherd's Purse *(Capsella bursa-pastoris)*	Whole Plant
Slippery Elm *(Ulmus rubra)*	Inner bark
Spearmint *(Mentha spicata)*	Leaves & flowers
Yarrow *(Achillea millefolium)*	Whole flowering plant

Herbal Preparations

Herbs are **essential** to have on hand in any **survival situation,** especially when medical facilities are unavailable or unreliable. It is important, therefore, to learn how to preserve herbs and make many of the basic herb formulas, not only for **emergencies,** but to have on hand for everyday use. As you learn to gather, preserve and use the familiar herbs around you, you will gain knowledge and appreciation for their marvelous **healing qualities** and for the **Creator.**

Most herbs, if gathered and dried properly, and stored in a cool, dry place, will keep for many years (Although their medicinal value depreciates each year). Ideally, herbs should be used fresh, but since this isn't always possible (especially during winter months) the following herb preparations are described.

Teas (Infusion)

An infusion is made from the flowers and/or leaves of fresh or dried herbs. (Herbs may be whole, cut or powdered).

Directions: Bring to a boil 1 or more cups of water and add 1 tbsp. fresh herb or 1 tsp. dried herb to each cup of water. Remove from heat and let steep 10-20 minutes. (For extra strength, steep longer.) Strain and add honey to sweeten, if desired. Remember: **never boil your herbs.**

Teas (Decoction)

A decoction is made from the bark, inner bark, or roots of trees and herbs.

Directions: Bring to a boil 1 or more cups of water. Add 2 tbsp. cut-up root or bark to each cup of water. Gently boil for 5-10 minutes, then remove from heat and let steep 25-35 minutes. Strain and repeat the process with the same herbs. Add both liquids together and add honey to sweeten, if desired.

Herbal Enemas

An enema bag should always be included in any survival kit. Always keep one on hand in the home or when traveling.

Directions: Pour 1-2 qts. lukewarm herbal tea (Catnip, Yarrow, Horsetail, etc.) into a clean enema bag. Retain liquid as long as possible while massaging bowel area through abdomen. (Lying on a slant board is ideal.) Evacuate liquid when pressure or discomfort occurs.

Fomentation (Compress)

Directions: Take a piece of natural cloth (cotton, wool, etc.) and dip into warm infusion or decoction (teas). Wring it out just enough so it isn't dripping. Place over desired area and secure with a piece of plastic and tape.

Poultice

Directions: A poultice can be made by heating fresh or dried herbs in water and straining, placing the herbs in a natural cloth and securing with a piece of plastic and tape over desired area. Or, a poultice can be made by chewing, bruising or chopping fresh herbs and placing them directly on skin or placing in a wet, natural cloth and securing with a piece of plastic and tape over desired area.

Bolus

A bolus is used internally as a poultice for the vagina or rectal area.

Directions: Mix enough powdered herb with olive oil to the consistency of bread dough. Roll into a long roll the diameter of your smallest finger. Cut into one inch lengths and freeze until ready to use. Insert one or two at night before going to bed. Rinse out with douche or enema in the morning.

Tinctures (Extracts)

Tinctures are much more concentrated than teas and can be easily assimilated.

Directions: Mix 8 oz. dried/cut herb, or 4 oz. powdered herb to 16 oz. (1 pint) of alcohol. (Alcohol must be at least 80 proof. Vodka or Everclear brands are recommended.) Age for 14 days, shaking bottle 2-4 times a day, gently mixing well. (Some believe it's best to go by the phases of the moon, starting on the new moon and ending on the full moon.) After 14 days, strain and pour into amber glass bottles and cap tightly. Tinctures will keep this way indefinitely with little loss of potency. It is the ideal way to store herbs if you want them to last. If you don't want to ingest the alcohol, simply add your tincture dose to a cup of hot water. The alcohol wit dissipate into the air.

Herbal Oils

Directions: Cover desired amount of fresh or dried herbs with olive oil. Keep in warm place for 2-3 weeks or warm on low heat for 1½-2 hours, stirring occasionally. (Do not boil.) Strain and press oil from herbs. Store in refrigerator to keep from spoiling. (Add vegetable glycerine to keep for longer periods.)

Ointment

Directions: Cover desired amount of herbs with olive oil (tallow or lanolin can be used if you don't mind using animal products.) Gently warm on low heat for 1½-2 hours, stirring occasionally. Strain and add melted beeswax to reach desired consistency (I generally use 1 tbsp. beeswax to 1 oz. Olive oil.) An ointment of coconut oil or cocoa butter can be made simply by heating herbs in melted oil and straining. This ointment must be kept cool (Not exceeding 80°F) or it will melt.

Herbal Baths

The skin is the largest organ of the body. It eliminates a least 2 lbs. of toxins a day. Therefore it is an extremely important organ for eliminating wastes and toxins from the body and promoting good health. Herbal baths help to open up skin pores and promote perspiration which assists the body during fevers, eliminating heavy metals and poison: from the body.

Directions: Before bathing, brush skin with a natural bristle brush or loofah sponge. Drink herbal teas (Catnip, Yarrow, Nettle) while bathing.

Ginger Bath: Add 2-4 tbsp. powdered Ginger to warm bath water. Use for fevers, colds/flu, sore muscles, or whatever ails you.

Herbal Sitz Bath: Soak 4-8 oz. of dried herbs (Nettle, Yarrow, Horsetail, etc.) or a gallon-size container full of fresh herbs in cold water for a least 12 hours. Heat up without boiling. Strain and add to bath water. (Soak in it for 20-30 minutes.) This is great for pregnant mothers and to speed recovery in any illness.

Mineral Bath: (For radiation or heavy metal poisoning.) Add 2 lbs. Epsom Salts to hot bath water. Soak for 1 hour and then drain. Add 2 lbs. baking soda to hot bath water and soak for 1 hour. Drink Bugleweed/Yellow Dock Combination and Yarrow teas while in the bath.

Herbal Footbath: Same as Herbal Baths but use half as much herbs.

*Use fresh herbs whenever possible as they have more strength than dried herbs.

Herbal Sources of Minerals

(Found in this book "**In the Woods**")

Iron: Yellow Dock, Nettles, Mullein, Pennyroyal, Chickweed, Burdock, Comfrey, Red Clover, Dandelion, Watercress, Alfalfa, Cayenne, Echinacea, Horsetail, Ginger, Garlic, Rose Hips, Yarrow, Sage, Peppermint, Slippery Elm, Oak Bark, Black Cohosh.

Calcium: Horsetail, Nettles, Watercress, Shepherd's Purse, Dandelion, Alfalfa, Red Clover, Red Raspberry leaf, Plantain, Chickweed, Comfrey, Garlic, Rose Hips, Slippery Elm, Peppermint, Oak Bark, Ginger, Oregon Grape Root, Black Cohosh, Mullein.

Potassium: Plantain, Peppermint, Yarrow, Nettles, Dandelion, Watercress, Comfrey, Alfalfa, Rose Hips, Mullein, White Oak Bar, Red Raspberry, Echinacea, Slippery Elm, Catnip, Chickweed, Red Clover, Black Cohosh, Sage.

Sodium: Alfalfa, Catnip, White Oak Bark, Horsetail, Lobelia, Ginger, Dandelion, Rose Hips, Slippery Elm, Pennyroyal, Chickweed, Comfrey, Sage, Mullein, Nettles.

Magnesium: Mullein, Dandelion, Black Cohosh, Alfalfa, Watercress, Garlic, Red Clover, Peppermint, Comfrey, Cayenne, Catnip, Ginger, Pennyroyal, Nettles, Chickweed, Burdock, Horsetail, Sage.

Silicon: Horsetail, Nettles, Dandelion, Mullein, Echinacea, Burdock, Pennyroyal, Chickweed, Black Cohosh, Garlic, Ginger.

Sulfer: Garlic, Alfalfa, White Oak Bark, Mullein, Peppermint, Dandelion, Burdock, Cayenne, Catnip, Comfrey, Lobelia, Echinacea.

Manganese: Watercress, Alfalfa, Yarrow, Horsetail, Catnip, Oregon Grape Root, Chickweed, Red Clover, Red Raspberry, Yellow Dock, Ginger, White Oak Bark, Mistletoe, Mullein, Peppermint.

Fluorine: Garlic, Watercress, Alfalfa.

Copper: Nettles, Horsetail, Alfalfa, Chickweed, Watercress, Burdock, Comfrey, Dandelion, Echinacea, Garlic, Lobelia, Peppermint, Yarrow, Slippery Elm, Red Clover, White Oak Bark.

Zinc: Watercress, Slippery Elm, Burdock, Chickweed, Comfrey, Dandelion, Garlic, Alfalfa, Black Cohosh, Cayenne, Echinacea, Horsetail, Sage, White Oak Bark, Nettles, Pennyroyal.

Iodine: Watercress.

Phosphorus: Alfalfa, Comfrey, Chickweed, Dandelion, Nettles, Red Raspberry leaf, Watercress, Black Cohosh, Oregon Grape Root, White Oak Bark, Ginger, Cayenne, Catnip, Horsetail, Garlic, Slippery Elm, Yellow Dock, Peppermint, Mullein, Red Clover.

Chromium: Nettles, Red Clover, Catnip, Yarrow, Horsetail, Black Cohosh, Chickweed, Echinacea, Garlic, Ginger, Horsetail, Pennyroyal.

Cobalt: Dandelion, Red Clover, Horsetail, Lobelia, White Oak Bark, Alfalfa, Cayenne, Echinacea, Nettles, Comfrey Mullein, Black Cohosh.

Selenium: Red Clover, Lobelia, Garlic, Slippery Elm, Alfalfa, Black Cohosh, Catnip, Comfrey, Peppermint, Chickweed, Echinacea, Pennyroyal.

Trace Minerals: Dandelion, Black Cohosh, Burdock, Alfalfa, Horsetail, Peppermint, Red Clover, Rose Hips, Yellow Dock, Lobelia, White Oak Bark.

Herbal Sources of Vitamins

(Found in this book "**In the Woods**")

Vitamin A (Retinol, Carotene): Alfalfa, Nettles, Mullein, Dandelion, Comfrey, Cayenne Yellow Dock, Watercress, Red Raspberry leaves, Lobelia, Black Cohosh, Burdock, Chickweed, Echinacea, Garlic, Ginger, Red Clover, Peppermint, Rose Hips, Yarrow.

Vitamin B1 (Thiamine): Catnip, Rose Hips, Dandelion, Red Clover, Red Raspberry leaves, Slippery Elm, Alfalfa, Burdock, Cayenne, Chickweed, Garlic, Mullein, Yellow Dock, Black Cohosh.

Vitamin B2 (Riboflavin): Dandelion, Rose Hips, Yellow Dock, Alfalfa, Catnip, Cayenne, Ginger, Red Clover, Chickweed, Echinacea, Horsetail, Black Cohosh.

Vitamin B3 (Niacin): Alfalfa, Dandelion, Slippery Elm, Red Raspberry, Burdock Seed and Root, Ginger, Red Clover, Mullein, Rose Hips, Cayenne, Chickweed, Black Cohosh.

Vitamin B5 (Pantothenic Acid): Alfalfa, Catnip, Black Cohosh, Burdock, Horsetail, Ginger, Mullein, Red Clover, Dandelion, Cayenne, Chickweed,

Vitamin B6 (Pyridoxine): Red Clover, Chickweed, Catnip, Alfalfa, Burdock, Cayenne, Ginger, Dandelion, Mullein.

Vitamin B9 (Folic Acid): Red Clover, Mullein, Catnip, Alfalfa, Burdock, Cayenne, Chickweed, Dandelion, Ginger.

Vitamin B12 (Cobalamin): Catnip, Alfalfa, Comfrey, Burdock, Dandelion, Ginger, Mullein, Red Clover, White Oak Bark, Chickweed, Cayenne.

Vitamin B15 (Pangamic Acid): Black Walnut. Vitamin B17 (Laetrile): Red Clover, Alfalfa.

Chorline: Alfalfa, Catnip, Mullein, Red Clover, Chickweed, Burdock, Dandelion, Cayenne.

Inositol: Red Clover, Mullein, Dandelion, Catnip, Alfalfa, Burdock, Cayenne, Chickweed.

Paba (Para-Amino Benzoic Acid): Horsetail, Mullein,

Red Clover, Catnip, Chickweed, Dandelion, Alfalfa, Burdock, Cayenne, Ginger.

Vitamin C (Ascorbic Acid): Red Clover, Burdock, Nettles, Mullein, Comfrey, Plantain, Alfalfa, Cayenne, Pine Needles, Catnip, Burdock, Black Cohosh, Chickweed, Garlic, Ginger, Dandelion, Echinacea, Peppermint, Red Clover, Yarrow, Rose Hips, Yellow Dock, Oregon Grape Root, Lobelia.

Vitamin D (Calciferol, Viosterol, Ergosterol): Nettles, Alfalfa, Chickweed, Rose Hips, Mullein, Red Raspberry leaf. Vitamin E (Tocopherol): Dandelion, Watercress, Alfalfa, Rose Hips, Red Raspberry leaf, Comfrey, Burdock, Echinacea, Slippery Elm, Yarrow.

Vitamin F (Linoleic Acid): Slippery Elm, Yarrow, Red Raspberry leaf. Vitamin H (Biotin): Red Clover, Ginger, Mullein, Cayenne, Dandelion, Alfalfa, Burdock, Chickweed, Catnip.

Vitamin K (Menadine): Nettles, Alfalfa, Horsetail, Yarrow, Slippery Elm.

Vitamin P (Bioflavanoids): Rose Hips, Cayenne, Burdock, Dandelion, Red Clover, Slippery Elm.

PART IV

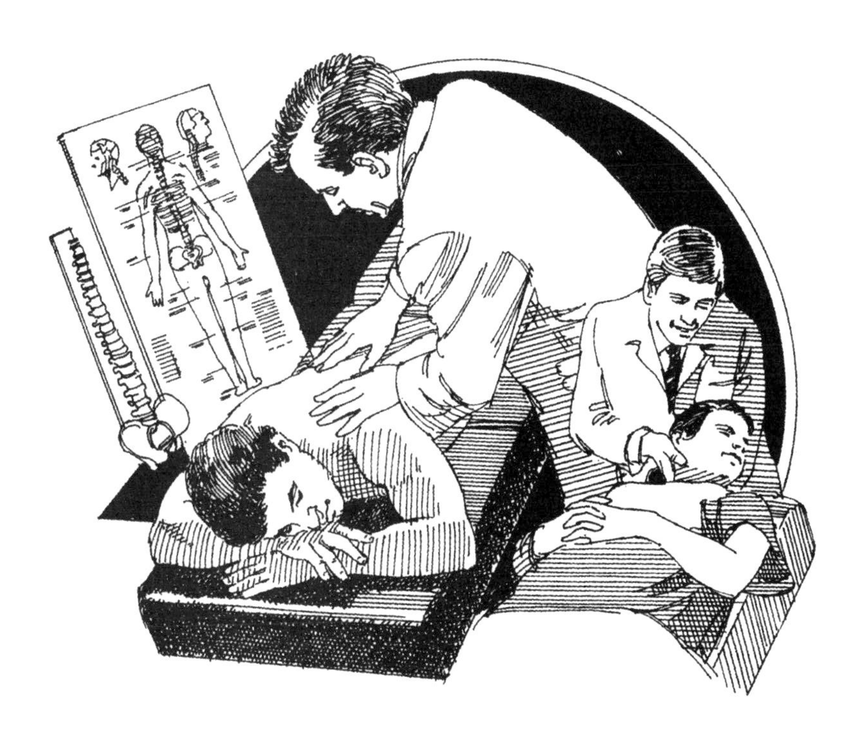

But pray ye that your flight be not in winter, neither on the Sabbath day. For then shall be great tribulation, such as was not seen since the beginning of the world to this time, no, nor ever shall be.

—St. Matthew (24:20-21)

PART IV

Appendix

Bleeding (Severe)

If severe bleeding from the head or extremities is not controlled within 10 minutes after using gauze pads and firm pressure over wound, add more gauze pads and apply more pressure using **"pressure points"** on major arteries (blood vessels carrying blood from the heart to the body). Apply pressure with thumb and fingers to the major artery supplying blood to the wounded area.

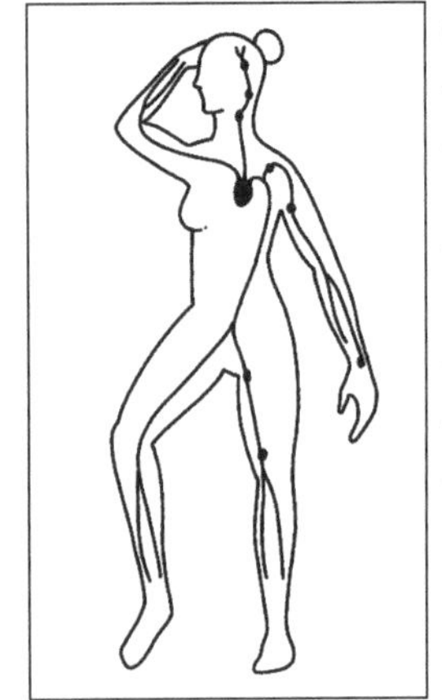

Also, to help control bleeding along with holding pressure points, **elevate** the **limb** that is involved. (Caution: If there is a fracture to the limb, this procedure is inadvisable.)

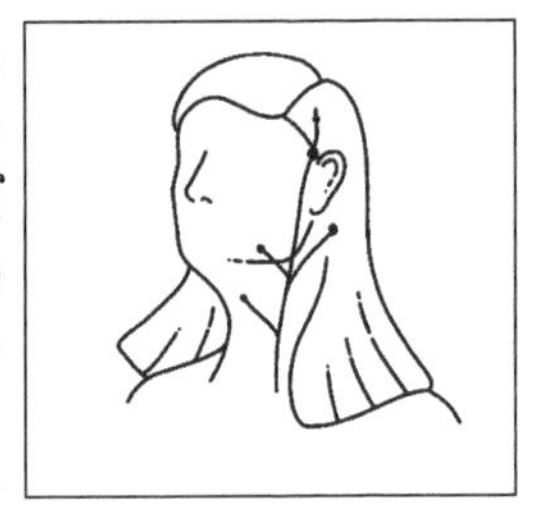

If severe bleeding continues after use of above procedures, with blood spurting from wound with each heart beat, the use of a **tourniquet** may be required to save a life (especially in cases where the person has lost a limb). This should be used as a **last resort** as it may require the **sacrifice of the limb.**

To apply tourniquet: Wrap cloth or bandage several inches wide above the wound and tie a half knot. Place a rigid piece of wood on the half-knot and tie one or two additional knots on top. Twist the stick to tighten the tourniquet until bleeding stops. Secure ends of stick with additional strips of cloth. Leave on for half an hour, then loosen. If bleeding has stopped, tourniquet can be removed. If not, retighten to stop bleeding.

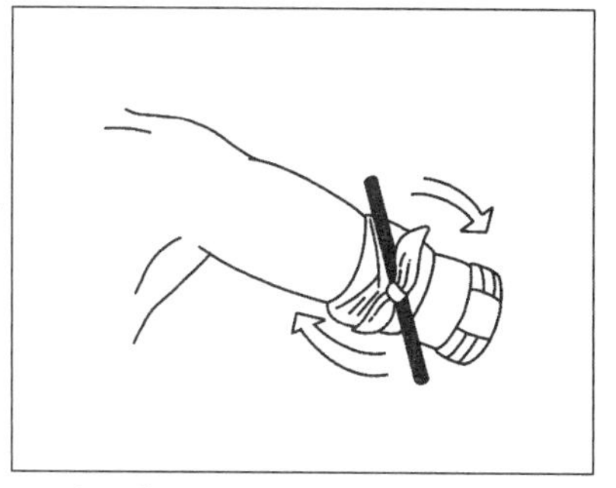

Application of Tourniquet

Breathing (Artificial Respiration)

Cessation of **breathing** is a **medical emergency** requiring immediate treatment. The following steps should be taken **immediately:**

(1) Make sure the air passageway is cleared of any obstructions. Remove any foreign objects from mouth or nose.
(2) Tip the person's head back while extending neck to maximize airway. (Do not overextend neck or tip head back if neck is injured.)
(3) Pinch nostrils together and rest palm of hand on forehead.
(4) Take a deep breath and seal your lips tightly over mouth.
(5) Blow deep, quick breaths, releasing mouth after each breath. The person's chest should noticeably expand during this procedure.
(6) Continue breathing into person (12 breaths per minute) until person is breathing on their own. NOTE: If there is no response, check airway again for foreign objects. If pulse cannot be found, administer CPR (See instructions for CPR in this appendix).

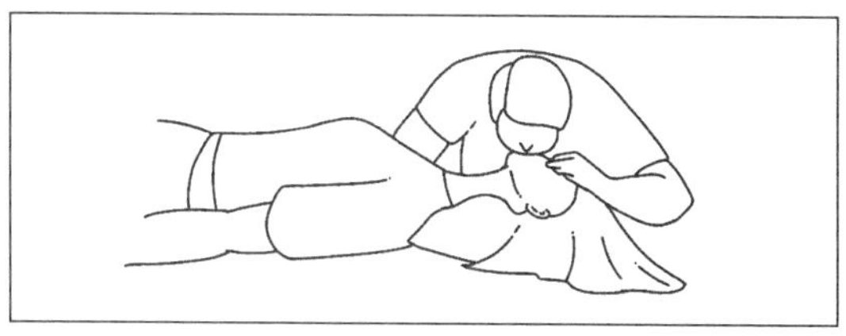

Position for Artificial Respiration

Choking (Heimlich Maneuver)

A leading cause of **death** in the home is obstruction of the throat or air passage by a foreign object (or choking). Most of these deaths occur among children under the age of 4 who either place objects in their mouths or are given food too large or hard for them to eat.

If someone shows signs of choking—can't speak, talk or breath, clutches throat, face turns blue, the **following** maneuver should be used **immediately:**

Stand person up and wrap arms around them from behind. Make fist with one hand, covering it with the other. Place top of

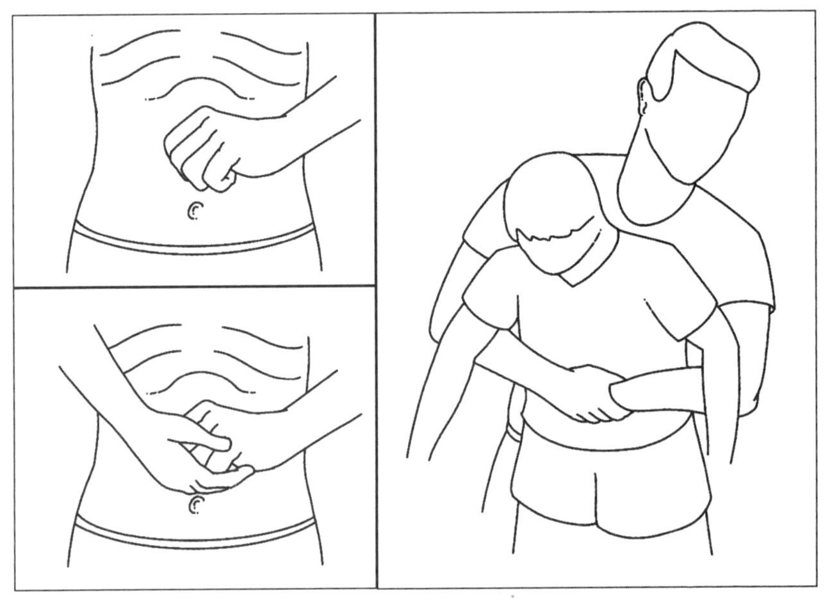

The Heimlich Maneuver (Abdominal Thrusts)

the fist just above the person's navel but under rib cage. Thrust fist upward and back into person's abdomen. Repeat four times or until object is dislodged. If this doesn't work, place person on side and, using the heel of your hand, hit sharply on spine between shoulder blades.

CPR (Cardio-pulmonary Resuscitation)

CPR should only be **administered** when **breathing** has **stopped** and there is **no pulse.** Check neck artery carefully as pulse may be weak. If there is a heartbeat but no sign of breathing, see Breathing (Artificial Respiration) in this appendix.

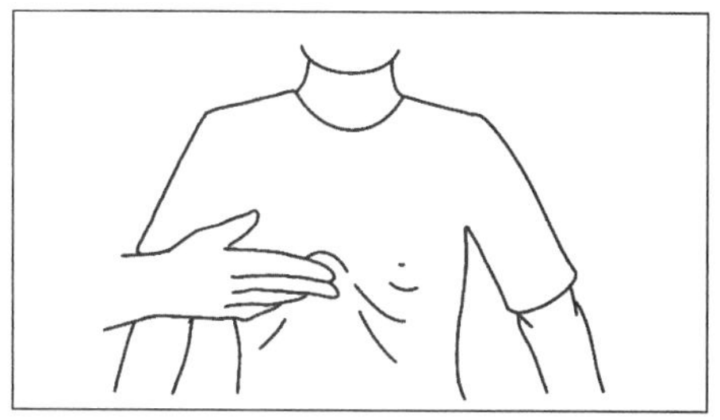

If no pulse, use the following procedure for **CPR:**

(1) Place index and middle finger on center of lower breastbone.

(2) Place heel of other hand next to and touching the index finger.

(3) For adults and children over 80 pounds only, place heel of the first hand on the person's lower breastbone. Clasp fingers and bend those of lower hand back. **For children under 80 pounds, use heel of only one hand.**

(4) Lean directly over the person and straighten your arm(s). Use straight-down pressure through arm or arms to push breastbone against heart. **For an adult,** depress breastbone 1½" to 2"; **for a child,** ¾" to 1½".

(5) The compression/relaxation combination is performed at a rate of 80 times per minute. Release pressure completely between strokes.

(6) After 30 compressions, breathe twice into mouth. Repeat the 30 to 2 cycle until pulse is felt or person revives. If there is a pulse, but no breathing, continue

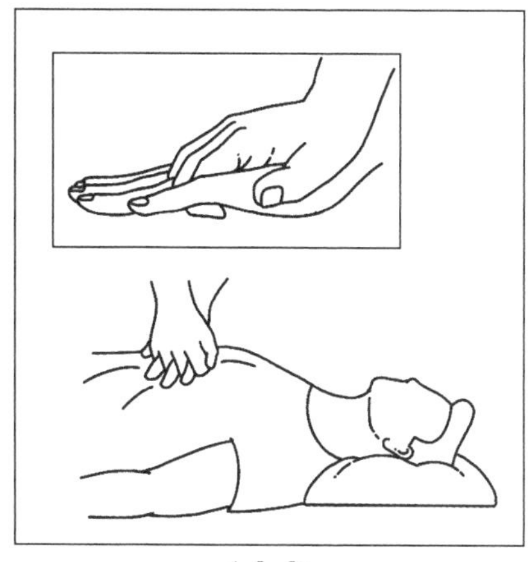

Adult

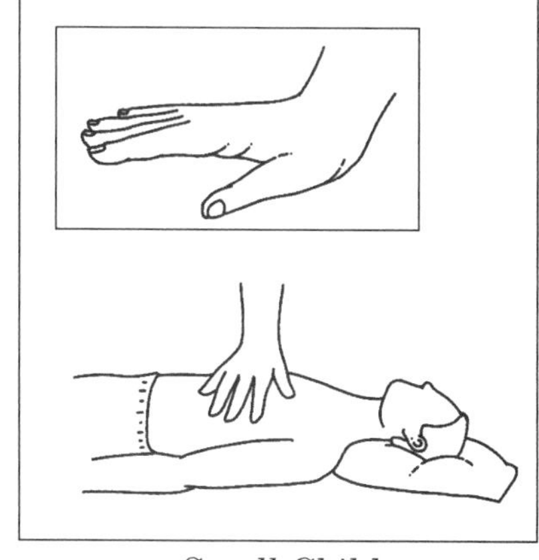

Small Child

with artificial ventilation only at a rate of 12 breaths per minute. (See breathing (Artificial Respiration) in this appendix.)

Frostbite

Usually the most common freezing of the tissues exposed to the elements are the face, hands and feet. Watch for possible pain in the early stages. The exposed part will become numb and turn white or grayish-yellow in progressed stages and blisters may appear on the skin. (Do not break blisters).

The best thing for frostbite is prevention. Always bring extra clothing when hiking in cold weather and make sure hands and feet are kept dry and covered. (Use any type insulation . available, dry grass stuffed in gloves and boots works well, in an emergency.)

If frostbite is suspected:

(1) Find shelter for the person, get them out of the elements. Take off any wet clothing. Wrap entire body in blankets, sleeping bags, coats, etc., to prevent hypothermia

(2) Do not rub frostbitten areas, as it can cause further damage. Also, refreezing after rewarming can cause serious damage and should be avoided at all costs. A person can walk many miles on frozen feet, but as soon as the rewarming takes place, the person will be laid up and unable to walk until healing takes place. So make sure if you can't get to a hospital, that you can stay in one place until healed after rewarming of frostbitten areas.

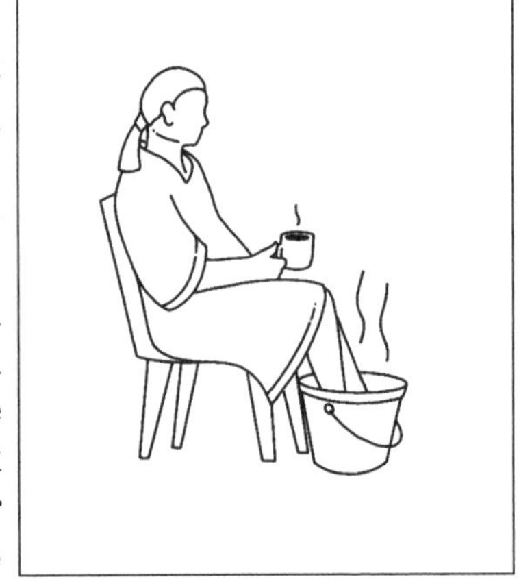

(3) If in a remote area with no chance of getting to a hospital, warm up some water (104°-108°F, check by putting hand in water and feel to where it is comfortably warm), add 1 tbsp. **Ginger** powder and 2 tbsp. **Cayenne** powder to 2 gallons.

Soak frostbitten area in warm water solution for at least an hour or until frostbitten area becomes flushed. (If feet are involved, do not allow person to walk.)

(4) During the rewarming, and afterwards, drink Nettle, Horsetail, Catnip, Mint tea or other warm liquids. Take 1 dropper Cayenne Tincture* under tongue.

(5) Dry off frostbitten area very gently without rubbing Separate toes or finger by placing rolled gauze or clean cloth between them. Raise affected parts and keep from Contact with bedclothes or the materials. Apply **Complete Tissue and Bone Ointment** after pain is gone. Drink Nettle and Horsetail tea, 4 cups a day.

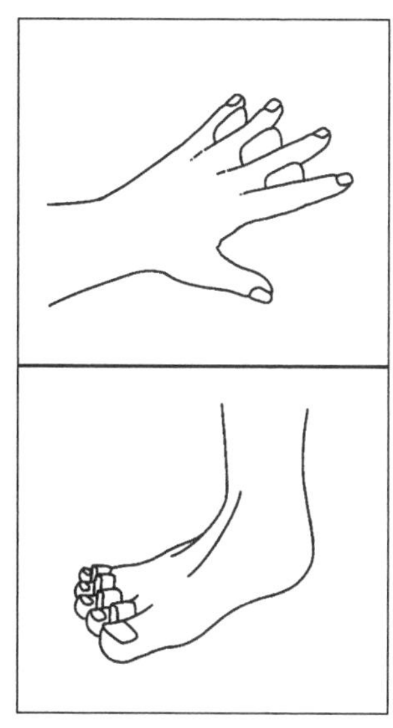

IN THE WOODS: Same 8 above, except you can us Mistletoe or Calamus root (if you can find them) instead of Ginger and Cayenne. Both must be brought to a boil and steeped long as possible. (Overnight . best, but not always practical. Use 1 handful of each per gallon of water. Strain before using. Also, the inner bark of Birch, Willow, Oak, Poplar, Larch, Aspen can be USE as a tea to promote healing (NOTE: As frostbite occurs in winter, fresh herbs would not be available. It is high recommended to carry Cayenne, Ginger and other preserved herbs with you in case of frostbite or other emergencies.)

Heatstroke

The body can suffer a number of reactions when exposed to excessive heat. The elderly, chronic invalid very young, alcoholics, and people who are over weight are the most likely to suffer from heat stroke. Heatstroke may happen with strenuous activity when there is high temperatures. **Always drink plenty of liquids** while doing strenuous activities in hot weather. Heat stroke (body temperature of 105°-106°F) is a very serious, medical emergency.

Treatment: Body temperature must be lowered **immediately.** Immerse patient in cold-water bath, stream, or lake with clothing removed. Or use a sponge or cloth soaked in cold water to cool the skin. Check temperature every 5-10 minutes until it drops to 100°-102°F. (If no thermometer, until person feels normal to touch. **Do not overchill.**)

During and after cooling down process, have person lie or sit in a shaded area, out of the sun. If temperature begins to rise again, repeat the cooling process. If the person gets chilled, cover with blanket.

Symptoms of heat stroke are very high body temperature (104°-106°F), absence of sweating, skin is hot, red and dry. Person may be in a stupor or perhaps unconscious.

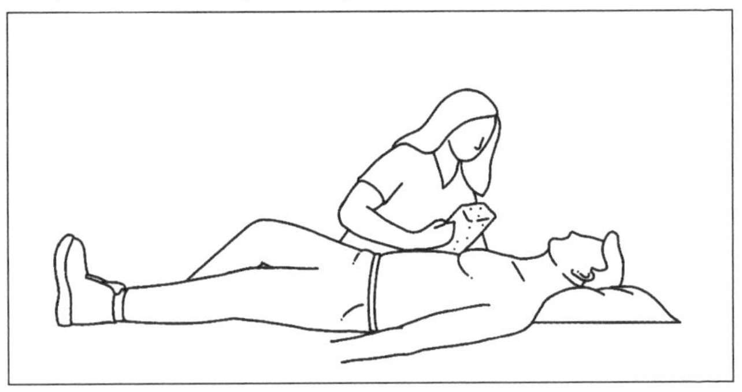

CAUTION: Do not give the person any stimulants (alcohol, coffee, tea, etc.).

After the body temperature is lowered (102°F) and person is no longer in a stupor, drink 1-2 cups of celery juice. If this is not available, drink 4-8 cups of cool water with ½ tsp. salt added.

IN THE WOODS: Same as above (where applicable). \
After temperature returns to normal, drink Horsetail, Alfalfa, Nettle tea, 3-4 cups a day to build strength.

Hemorrhage (Heavy Bleeding)

Stopping blood loss takes priority over any other treatment except cessation of breathing or heart beat, which needs to be treated together with CPR.

Almost all bleeding can be controlled by covering wound

with **Cayenne** powder and applying direct pressure on the wound with sterile 3x3" or 4x4" gauze dressings from the First Aid Kit* over the wound. Apply constant firm pressure for 10-15 minutes or until bleeding stops. **Give Cayenne Tincture.** Dose: 1 dropper every 5-10 min. Then bandage with clear gauze and tape.

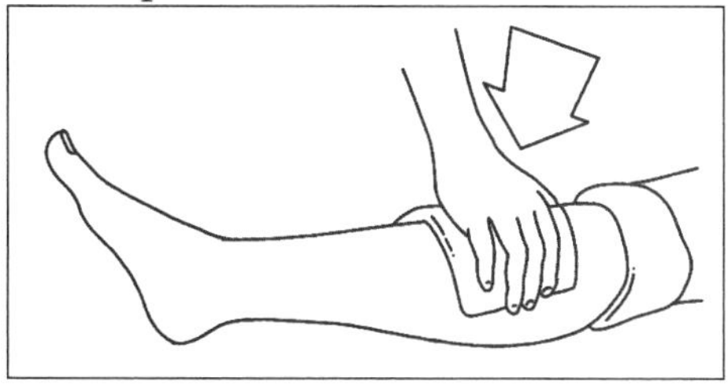

If the person has lost a lot of blood, treat for shock (See Shock). Keep person warm, calm and reassured.

Apply firm pressure over bleeding wound

IN THE WOODS: Use Hemostatic Herbs (Herbs that stop bleeding) both internally and externally (Horsetail, Mistletoe, Stinging Nettle, Shepherd's Purse, Yarrow, etc. Apply pressure as described above. (For more detailed information, see Bleeding (Severe), in this appendix.)

Hypothermia

The number one concept in the woods for survival is to stay **calm, dry** and **warm.** With most wilderness medical problems, prevention is always more important than treatment. If you do become cold, wet or exhausted, find or make a shelter where you are out of the harsh elements.

Two of the greatest dangers of hypothermia are physical exhaustion and wet clothing. People who are the most likely to succumb to hypothermia are those of a thin body type (usually male) who lack sufficient body fat to help insulate against the cold.

Symptoms of hypothermia are fatigue, shivering, goose pimples, hallucinations, disorientation, drowsiness, slurreld speech, and low body temperature. (91°-98°F). If any of these symptoms occur, find shelter immediately out of the elements, and begin treatment for hypothermia. With hypothermia, **death** can occur in a surprisingly short time (few hours), even when the temperatures are not freezing but it is windy and the person is wet, malnourished, or not clothed properly. Hypothermia is common when there are head injuries, loss of blood, a fracture and the person is immobilized in cold weather, and in shock.

Treatment: For mild hypothermia, (body temperature of 95°F or higher) make sure the person is in dry clothing, adding more clothes, blankets, or sleeping bags to keep warm. Administer 1 dropper of **Cayenne Tincture** and **Nettle Tincture** and give warm teas made from **Ginger,** Nettle, Yarrow, sweetened with honey. (Hot soup or drinks can be used if herbs are not available.) Keep person out of wind and elements in a proper shelter. Apply **Cayenne Heat Ointment** to chest, neck, back, feet and hands. (Avoid eyes and pubic area)

For moderate hypothermia, (body temperature 90° -94°F). Treat the same as mild hypothermia except additional heat needs to be provided as fast as possible to the person's body without burning them. One of the best ways is to get one or two persons that are warm into a sleeping bag (like a cocoon) with the victim, skin to skin contact. This will bring up the victim's body core temperature quickly and safely (Hot water bottles, warm baths, warm stones, or any other **safe** heat source can also be used.)

If you don't have a thermometer and can't tell the severity of the hypothermia, treat as if moderate to severe. (Don't give teas if unconscious.)

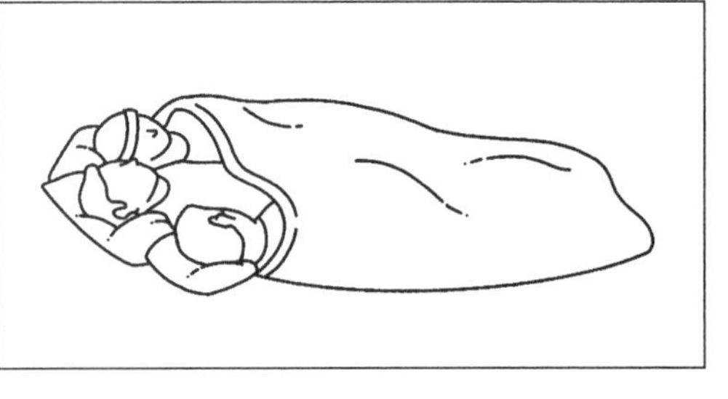

When the shivering stops (when the body temperature is rising), it is a good sign. But if it stops when the body temperature is falling, it is a bad sign. (Shivering is the body's way of producing heat.)

Symptoms of severe hypothermia: Body temperature is 80°-90°F, muscles rigid, gross incoordination occurs; mental activity dulls; unresponsiveness (coma), pulse an respiration slows down. Body temperature below 80°F is life threatening, with irregularities of the heart. Few people survive body temperatures below 75°F. These symptoms are something to watch for, but in order to accurately determine body core temperature, a thermometer capable of reading from 75° to 105° is necessary.

The important thing to remember in all cases of hypothermia is that the body's central core (the torso) is warmed **first** before warming the extremities. It is dangerous to warm the extremities if the central part of the body is not being heated In severe hypothermia, use your own judgement on how much **Cayenne Tincture** or **Shepherd's Purse Tincture** to give. (Personally, I would give whatever it takes to get the body core temperature up and improvement in circulation)

In severe cases of hypothermia, do not treat victim if hospitalization is available. There are sophisticate treatments to warm these potentially lethal cases that hospitals are equipped for.

Insect Bites (Poisonous)

Treat similarly as for poisonous snake bites.

(1) Have person lie down and remain calm; cover them with a blanket, coat, sleeping bag, etc.

(2) Administer
Echinacea Tincture.
Dose: ½ to 1 oz. at first; next day, ½ dropper 3 times a day until healed
Plantain Tincture
Dose: 10-20 drops 3 times a day.
Yarrow Tincture
Dose: 10-20 drops 2 times a day.
Black Cohosh Tincture
Dose: 5-10 drops 2 times a day.

(3) If the bite took place within 30 minutes, tie a piece of cloth 2-5 inches above bite (not on a joint). Tie snugly, but not too tight. Be able to slip a finger under it.

(4) Wash bite area with clean water and soap. Apply cold compress while you are making a poultice or fomentation from Plantain, then apply it over bite area. Leave on until redness or swelling is gone.

(5) If nervous problems occur (fits, depression, crying, short tempered), use **Ear & Nerve Tincture.** Dose:

15-20 drops 3 times a day. Also for nervous problems, and/or leg cramps, fevers, chills, use **Horsetail Tincture.** Dose: 20 drops 3 times a day

IN THE WOODS: Same as above. Drink Plantain, Yarrow, Horsetail tea, 4-6 cups a day.

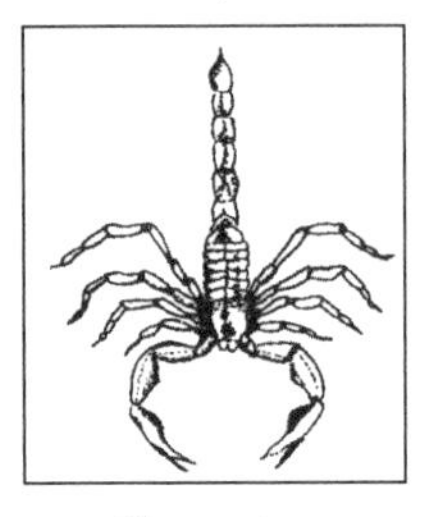

Scorpion

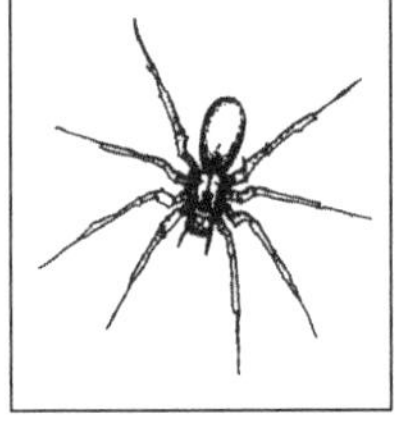

Brown Recluse Spider

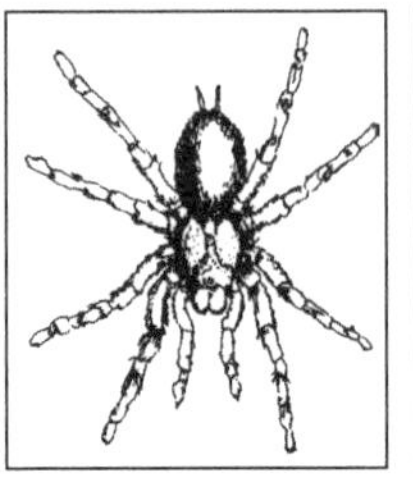

Tarantula

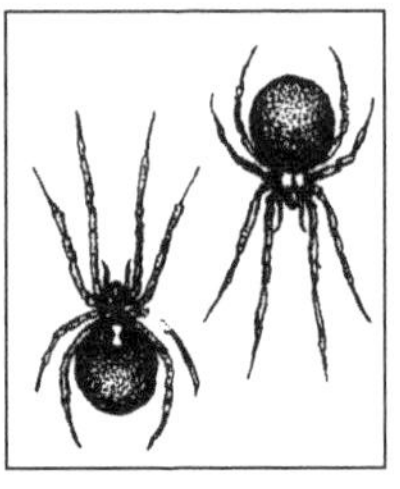

Black Widow Spider

AUTHOR'S NOTE: Lately, there has been an outbreak in the Arizona area of Brown Recluse Spider bites. With these bites, use Plantain fomentation over bite combined with **Echinacea Tincture** and Calendula Ointment until skin is healed.

Shock

Shock is a serious condition of a severe circulatory collapse. Most often it is caused by extreme blood loss, or traumatic injury without any blood loss.

The symptoms of shock to watch for are clamminess of skin, washed-out look, rapid weak pulse, low blood pressure, shallow rapid breathing, nausea and vomiting. Also watch for partial or complete loss of consciousness.

A state of shock can be induced by people with fear in a minor injury. In every accident follow as if shock could occur and treat as if it could occur even up to several hours later. Shock can be more serious than the injury.

If a person is conscious or unconscious:

(1) Administer 1 dropper of **Cayenne Tincture** under the tongue, followed by **Shepherd's Purse Tincture,** 1 dropper under tongue (to normalize circulation).

(2) Lie the person flat on their back, with legs and thighs elevated.

(3) Make sure the person is warm-replace any wet cloth-

ing. A person in mild shock can still produce body heat. A person in severe shock loses the ability to produce any body heat. When this happens, no amount of clothing will help to restore body heat. Hypothermia and irreversible shock then takes place, and the person can die. In severe shock, **external heat** needs to be applied. The best heat source is from another person, one or more, to come in contact skin to skin in sleeping bags (like a cocoon) with the person in shock. Internally, keep administering **Cayenne Tincture** and **Nettle Tincture** to improve circulation and produce internal heat. All future heat loss to the person in extreme shock should be avoided.

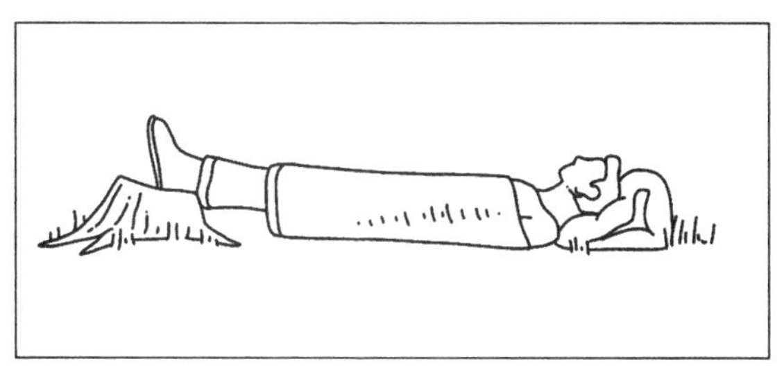

Position of person in shock

IN THE WOODS: Follow same procedure except have person drink Nettle and Shepherd's Purse tea, **if conscious.** (Do not administer tea if unconscious.)

Snakebite (Poisonous)

In cases of poisonous snakebite, time is of the essence.

(1) Have the person lie down and remain calm and still. Keep the bite below the level of the heart. Remove anything that would constrict (belts, rings, watches, bracelets, etc.).

(2) Administer **Echinacea Tincture.** Dose: 1-2 oz. **Plantain Tincture. Dose:** 25-30 drops every 5-10 minutes. **Yarrow Tincture. Dose:** 10-20 drops every 10-20 minutes. **Black Cohosh Tincture. Dose:** 10-20 drops 3 times a day (See Note).

(3) If you have a snakebite kit, apply suction to the bite without making an incision (Follow directions in kit).

(4) Wash bite area with clean water and soap. Apply

Xceptic Tincture over bite area, then apply Plantain poultice or fomentation over bite. If there is swelling, tie a piece of cloth or handkerchief snugly around the bitten limb, 3-5 inches above the bite. If swelling goes beyond this, apply a second band above this one, above the new swelling. Leave the first one on. (Make sure

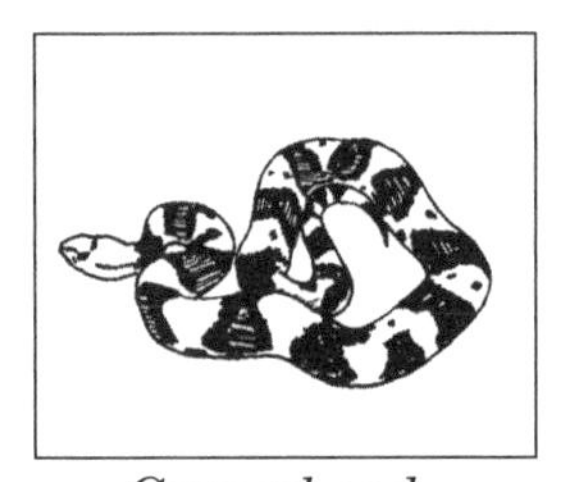

Copperhead
Copperheads in the U.S., when alarmed, vibrate their tails rapidly. Found in south-eastern U.S.

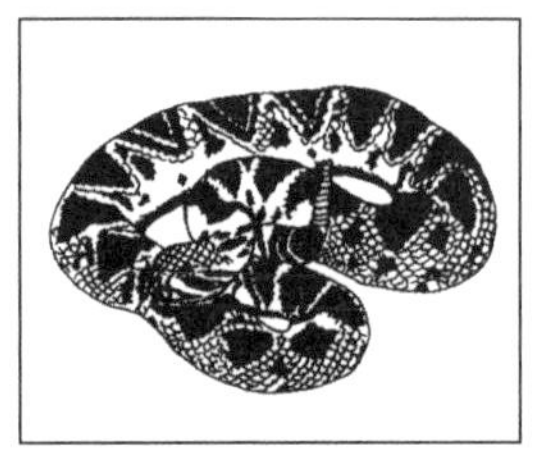

Rattlesnake
There are 14 different species found in the U.S. When alarmed the tails produce a sound like a rattle.

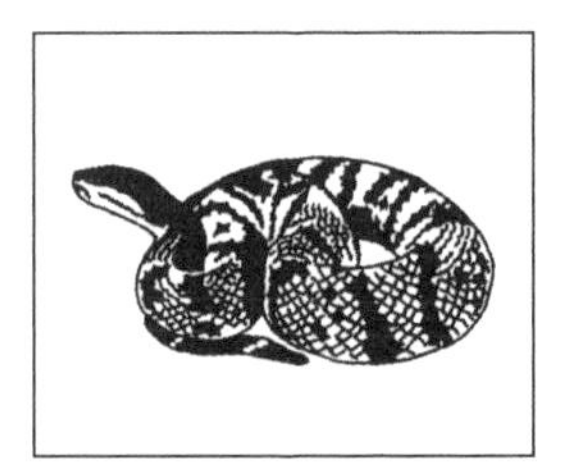

Cottonmouth
(Water Moccasin)
Found in Florida and Eastern parts. Cottonmouth is poisonous.

the band doesn't block arterial or venous circulation.)

IN THE WOODS: Same as above, except if you don't have tinctures on hand, have the victim chew and swallow as much Plantain as possible while venom is being suctioned out. If there is a third party, have them make a tea out of Plantain and Yarrow and drink as much as possible. (Caution: If you are alone or with one other person only, suction out venom first before making tea.) Apply Plantain poultice over bite area; change every 2-4 hours.

NOTE: Black Cohosh is a natural antidote for poisons in the system. It has the ability to neutralize the effects of rattlesnake bites, scorpion stings, and other poisons in the system.

Ticks

Ticks can cause a potential hazard to anyone in the outdoors because they can transmit many diseases. You should check often for ticks on clothing and exposed areas of your body, and especially the hair on your head and other body parts where they can hide. If you are with someone, have them check your

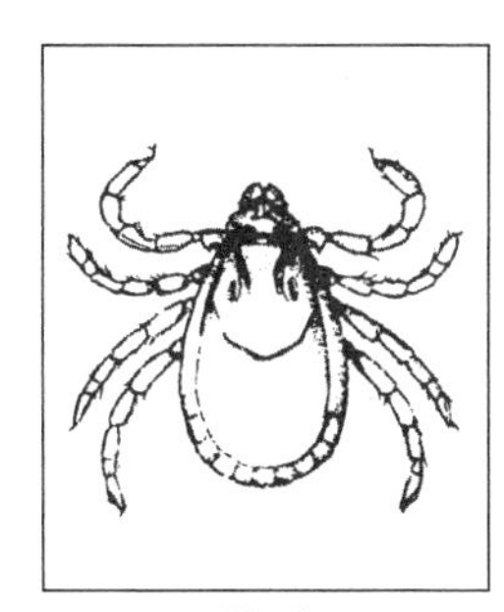

Tick
Brown/Gray in color. to 1/8-1/4" in length when fully grown. Flat and oval in shape, with dark colored head.

hair on your Tick head area about every 2-4 hours. (Run a comb or brush through your hair and then examine scalp carefully.) To help avoid ticks, use **Sen-Sei Balm** around wrist, ankles, neck and hairline.

Tick bites can cause generalized muscular weakness known as "tick paralysis." Any unexplained muscular weakness calls for a body search for ticks or tick bites.

In many locations throughout the U.S., ticks carry the Rocky Mountain Spotted Fever. (A sickness with the symptoms of a high fever, red-spotted rash.) Lyme disease is another more recent disease carried by ticks. (Symptoms are an expanding, circular, red rash where the tick bite is, flulike symptoms. A week to month later, serious heart, joint and nervous system abnormalities occur.) The tick that causes the Lyme disease is as small as a dot above an "i". It's hard to see, so do a careful search if symptoms appear.

Removal: Try to avoid direct contact with tick on removal. First, you can cover the tick completely with petroleum jelly or lip balm (Vaseline, Chapstick or heavy oil) to shut off its breathing pores. **Cayenne Heat Ointment** or **Sen-Sei Balm** works well also as insects don't like the essential oils in these two products. **If tick drops off,** wash the area well and apply **X-Ceptic Tincture** and **Garlic Oil.** Then apply **Black Ointment** to draw out any toxins left in the skin.

Internally, take Garlic Oil. Dose: 10-15 drops 3 times a day.

If tick doesn't drop off after 30-45 minutes with Vaseline, Chapstick or Herbal Balm applied, use clean tweezers to remove. Tweezer Removal: Turn tick on its back. Firmly but gently grasp near head at the point of attachment with tweezers and remove slowly. Make sure to remove entire tick, especially head and mouth parts.

If fever, use **Yarrow Tincture.**

Dose: 10-15 drops 4-6 times a day or until fever breaks.

IN THE WOODS: Use a hot Plantain, Yarrow poultice over tick and leave on for 15-30 minutes. If tick doesn't drop off, remove tick with tweezers (or scrape off with clean knife.) Wash area and apply Plantain poultice over area to heal and draw out any retained toxins. (Treat every tick bite as if you have been infected.) Drink Yarrow, Plantain, Nettle tea, 34 cups a day.

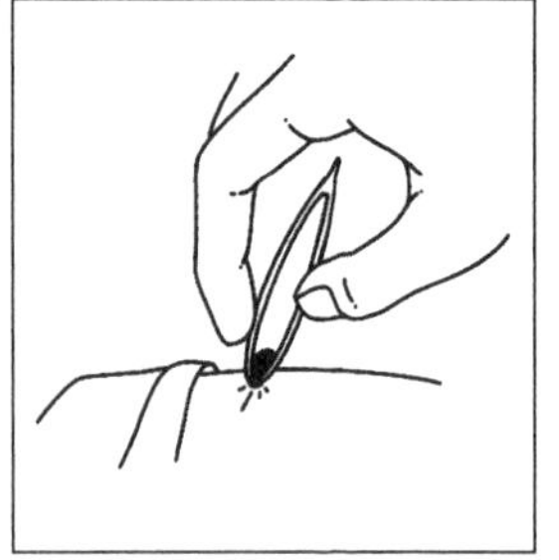

Wounds

Gently wash out wound with water that has been boiled or that you know is clean. If slightly bleeding (See **Bleeding** for Severe Bleeding), sprinkle with Cayenne* powder or apply Cayenne Tincture* to stop bleeding. Apply sterile dressing if wound is not gaping. If gaping, clean wound can be closed by the application of butterfly bandages. These are applied by adhering one side of bandage to one side of wound, the wound is pulled together, then the other side of bandage is taped to the other side of wound. (All wounds should be cleaned of all debris, dirt, rocks, twigs, etc., before closing the wound.) Apply **X-Ceptic Tincture** to wound to prevent infection. If bleeding continues, use Cayenne Tincture· or Powder* internally and externally.

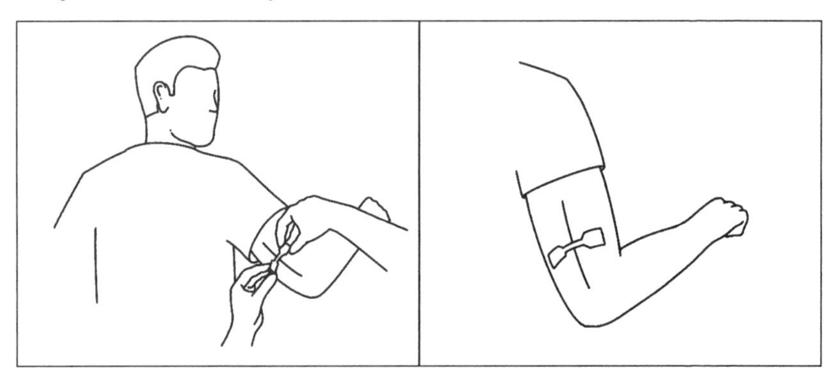

IN THE WOODS: Use Hemostatic Herbs (herbs that stop bleeding), both internally and externally-Horsetail, Mistletoe, Shepherd's Purse, Stinging Nettle, Yarrow. Drink as a tea, one or more, 2-4 cups a day. Use above herbs as a poultice over wound.

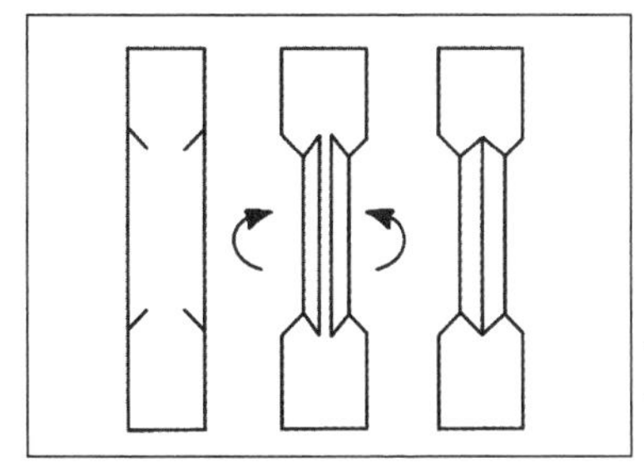

Making butterfly strips from adhesive tape when you have no butterfly bandages.
Adhesive tape cut 3½ inches long.
Make four cuts (slightly inward).

"And I heard another voice from Heaven saying, Come out of her my people, that ye be not partakers of her sins, and that ye receive not of her plagues."

—Revelation 18

Survival into the 21st Century

Observing animals in the wild, we notice that instinctively. they know when winter is coming ... and they **prepare.**

Observing the changes in the world, man-made and natural, it doesn't take a political genius or an earth scientist to realize that we are in a time of great transition . .. and we must prepare.

We must prepare ourselves for economic and political disasters as well as natural disasters, such as earthquakes, floods and famines, or we won't be counted as wise as the animals. If we stop and listen to the inner self (the spirit that moves in all things) it will tell us how to be prepared.

Personally, I am taking the following steps to prepare myself and family:

(1) Have at least a year's supply of food on hand. (The basics—grains, legumes, honey, spices, etc.)
(2) Have a year's supply of herbal medicines on hand and a basic knowledge of where to find them in nature and how to use them.
(3) Clothing for all occasions and all ages (If you have a large family like us).
(4) Non-hybrid seeds for a large garden for fresh food and seed storage.
(5) Tools and a basic knowledge of how to use them (For example: Construction tools, woodworking tools, looms, spinning wheels, potter's wheels, garden tools, etc.).
(6) "How to" books on everything!

Not only is it important that we try and save ourselves if disaster comes, but we should also be prepared to be of assistance to others who are less fortunate.

Healthy Food Storage

Yvonne L. Salcido MH

Today there is a myriad of ideas on food storage and many are lacking in sufficient nutrition. Who wants to just survive and be sick? The best plan for storage includes a high density of vitamins, mineral, proteins, and essential fats in the foods you store for optimum health. The following is a list of things I store.

Basic Storage for one person for one year:

300 lbs. Organic wheat (kamut, spelt)

155 lbs. A combination of organic grains (brown rice, buckwheat, oat groats, millet, quinoa, barley, corn, triticale, spelt, kamut etc.)

50 lbs. Raw nuts (25 lbs almonds, 5 lbs of additional favorites such as walnuts, cashews, pecans, pine nuts, etc.) Can use almonds to make nut milk.

20 lbs. Raw seeds (flax seeds, sunflower, pumpkin, sesame, chia, etc.)

75 lbs. Organic beans (pinto, black, red, white, garbanzo, lentils, mung beans, peas, soybeans, etc.)

60 lbs. Raw honey (also store some black strap molasses and agave – I use agave for special treats)

20 lbs. Oils (Olive oil, coconut and wheat germ oil)

10 lbs. Salt (vegetable, potassium based or sea salt)

60 lbs. Sprout mix (2 parts wheat, 1 part of the following: triticale, lentils, adzuki beans, mung beans, peas, then add 2 c. of fenugreek to the 60 lb. bucket)

5 lbs. Seed Sprout mix (alfalfa, radish and red clover)

Garden seeds (A good variety!)

Spices (You will want some different flavors)

Recipes for sprouting, live bread cracker, raw meals etc.

Herbal First Aid Kit

By Yvonne L. Salcido MH

An emergency kit should be in every home, car and place of business. Listed below are herbal formulas and products that I feel are essential for a first aid kit.

***Formulas By Dr. Christopher**

Cayenne	Extract, powder, and ointment
X-Ceptic*	Extract
Sensei*	Ointment
Lobelia	Extract
Super Garlic Immune*	Extract
Echinacea	Extract
Plantain	Ointment
Ginger	Powder, or capsules
X-INFX*	Capsules or powder
Oil of Oregano	Essential oil
Complete Tissue & Bone*	Capsules or powder, cut, & ointment
Nettle	Capsules or powder
Immucalm*	Capsules or powder or Marshmallow & Astragalus powder
Burn Paste	Equal parts Comfrey powder (or Complete Tissue & Bone powder*), wheat germ oil, and raw honey
Garlic Oil*	Oil
Black Ointment*	ointment
Ear & Nerve Formula*	Extract/Tincture
Mullein/Lobelia Oil*	Oil
Herbal Eyebright*	Extract & eye cup
Anti-spasmotic*	Extract
Cleansing Formulas*	Capsules or Extracts—Lower Bowel*, Liver Gall Bladder*, Kidney*, and Bloodstream * Formulas
Super foods	Vital Herbs*, Jurassic Green*, Capsules or Powder,
Kiddie Formulas*	

Herbs for Year Supply

Yvonne L. Salcido MH

There is a definite peace that comes from having a ready supply of herbs on hand for a sudden illness or emergency. Recently I had a family member in another state call very sick. She wanted to know what she could do. She had nothing in the house on hand. What if the phones lines were down, even cell phones will not work in a major disaster. What if is she could not call to get advice? Most importantly is herbal education, this invaluable skill will bless many in circumstances that we can't predict. Look around us the world is having so many challenges from weather, earthquake, wars etc. Becoming self reliant is becoming critical.

Cayenne	extract powdered 1 lb. Ointment
Lobelia	extract cut 1 lb.
Garlic	whole cloves in vinegar or bulbs hung Garlic oil 2-2 oz. Super Garlic Immune* ANTI-PLAGUE
Complete Tissue & Bone* & COMFREY	powdered 1 lb. cut 1 lb. Ointment
Yarrow	cut 1 lb.
Brigham Tea	cut 1 lb.
Chaparral	cut 1 lb.
Mullein	cut 1 lb. Mullien oil
Nettle	powdered 1 lb.
X-INFX*	powder 1 lb.
Plantain	powdered 1 lb. Ointment 4 oz.

Red raspberry	cut 1 lb.
Echinacea	powdered 1 lb. & extract
X-Ceptic*	extract
Nerve Formula*	extract
Ear & Nerve Formula*	extract
Catnip	cut 1 lb.
Cleansing Herbs	Lower Bowel Formula*, Liver/ Gall Bladder Formula*, Kidney Formula*, & Blood Stream Formula*
Anti-spasmotic*	Extract
Nutritional Herbs	Vital Herbs*, Jurassic Green*, Kiddie Formulas*
Herbal Calcium extract*	
Slippery Elm	powder 1 lb.
Licorice Root	powder 1 lb.
Black Walnut	cut 1 lb. & extract
Pau de' Arco	cut 1 lb.
Ginger	powdered 1 lb.
Herbal Eyebright*	extract & eye cup
Chasteberry/	powdered 1 lb./ capsules
Mindtrac	
Oregano	oil
Black Ointment*	ointment

Additional items: Raw honey and wheat germ oil

*Formulas by Dr. Christopher

PART V

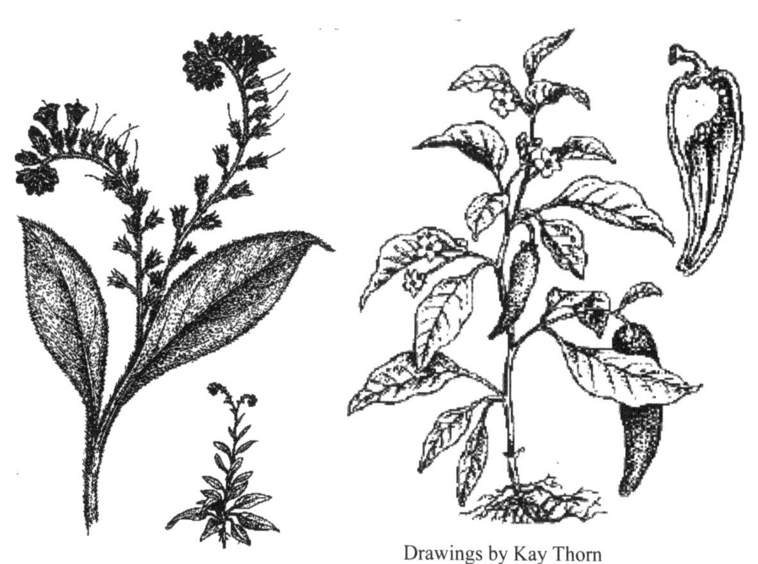

Drawings by Kay Thorn

Comfrey is one of the patriarchal herbs that I believe harkens back to the Garden of Eden. The Creator placed it on the Earth knowing that the human race was going to make a rough time of it and would need a universal salve for the wounds of war and accident.

Cayenne is one of the greatest herbs of all time—though it is also one of the most misunderstood and ridiculed. Every home should have a good supply.

— *Dr. John R. Christopher*

PART V

Comfrey and Cayenne

COMFREY — *Symphytum officinale*

FAMILY: Boraginaceae

COMMON NAMES:

- Comfrey
- knitbone
- healing herb
- bruisewort
- consound
- blackwort
- wallwort
- gum plant
- black root
- slippery root
- nipbone
- knitback
- yalluc (Saxon)
- Schwarzwurz (Ger)
- consuelda, sinfito (Spanish)

THERAPEUTIC ACTIONS:

- demulcent
- cell proliferant
- pectoral
- astringent
- nutritive
- tonic
- expectorant
- hemostatic
- alterative
- vulnerary
- mucilage
- styptic

MEDICINAL USES:

Anemia
Arthritis
Arthritic Fever
artherosclerosis
arthritis
asthma (including asphyxia)
Athlete's Foot
Bedsores
Bee Stings
Bites, Insect
Blood Pressure
bleeding
blood clots
bloody nose
blood pressure
blood thinner
Boils
Bones (bruised, broken)
Bowels (inflamed) backache
breathing
cancer
chicken pox / shingles
chilblains
chills
cholesterol (prevents absorption)
circulation
cleanses the circulatory system
cold hands and feet
colds / flu
colitis
congestion
constipation
coughs
counter irritant for chronic pain
cramps
creates endorphins
damaged tissue
debility
delirium treatments
diarrhea
digestion (aids)
dyspepsia
elimination (regulates)
emaciation
emesis
emphysema
fatigue
fever
frostbite
functional sluggishness
gangrene
gout
hair loss
headaches
heart attack
helps elasticity of arteries, veins, and caprilla
hemorrhaging (stops)
hemorrhoids
hiatal hernia
hypothermia
infection (prevents spread)
inflammation
intestinal mucus
kidney problems
lethargy
lowers cholesterol
lumbago
lung congestion
measles
memory
mouth sensitivity (increases)
nausea
neuralgia
night blindness
offensive breath
pain–blocks, numbs
pleurisy
pregnancy
pulse (strengthens)
rheumatism
saliva (increases)
scarlet fever
scurvy
shock
sore throats
stimulant
strep throat
stroke
tonsilitis
toothache
typhoid fever
ulcers
vomiting
yellow fever
wounds (speeds healing)

CAYENNE — *Capsicum annum*

Recommended dosage 1 tsp per cup of water
or 2 capsules three times a day

Bronchitis
Bruises
Bunion
Burns / Scalds
Cancer
Catarrah
Chicken Pox
Chilblains
Colitis
Conjunctivitis
Corn
Cough
Cuts / Grazes
Dermatitis
Diabetes
Diarrhea
Digestion
Duodenal Ulcers
Dysentery
Early Cellulitis
Eczema
Female debility
Fractures
Gangrene
Gastrojejunal Ulcer
Gout
Gravel
Gum Boils
Hay Fever
Heart Problems
Hemorrhage
Hemoptysis
Herpes
Horse Fly Bites
Ligaments (torn)
Leukorrhea
Mosquito Bites
Infected Thumb
Irritation
Inflammation
Joints (swelling)
Kidney (ulcerated)
Knee (swollen, sprained)
Lichen-Planus
Liver Trouble
Lung (inflamed, ulcerated)
Miners phthisis
Mole
Nettles
Nosebleed
Pancreatitis
Peripheral sores
Piles
Pinched Thigh
Pleurisy
Pneumonia
Psoriasis
Pulmonary T.B.
Rash
Rheumatism
Rib (cracked)
Ruptures
Scrofula
Shingles
Sinusitis
Skin Condition
Sore finger
Sore
Spot
Sprains
Stomach (inflamed)
Strains
Sunburn
Swellings
Thyroid
Tuberculosis
Ulcers
Urine (bloody)
Verruca
Wounds

References and Resources

Barlow, Max G. *From the Shepherd's Purse.* A Spice West Publication.

Bible. King James version.

Brown, Tom, Jr. *The tracker. The Search. The Vision. The Quest. Tom Brown's Field Guide to Wilderness Survival. Field Guide to Living with the Earth. Guide to Wild Edible Plants.* Berkley Books.

Christopher, John R. *School of Natural Healing. Childhood Diseases.* Christopher Publications.

Dadd, Debra Lynn. Nontoxic, *Natural and Earthwise.* Tarcher Publications.

Grieve, Mrs. M. *A Modern Herbal.* Penguin Books.

Heinerman, John, *Science of Herbal Medicine.* Bi-World.

Hutchens, Alma R. *Indian Herbology of North America.*

Keith, Velma and Monteen Gordon. *The How to Herb Book.* Mayfield Publications.

Kervran, Louis. *Biological Transmutations.* Swan House Publishing.

Kloss, Jethro. *Back to Eden.* Lifeline Books.

Kroeger, Hanna. *Instant Vitamin—Mineral Locator.*

Lust, John. *The Herb Book.* Bantam.

Mabey, Richard. *The New Age Herbalist.* Macmillan Publishing Company.

Mills, Charles F. *American Medicinal Plants.* Davis Press.

Moore, Michael. *Medicinal Plants of the Mountain West.* Museum of New Mexico Press.

Moulton, LeArta. *Herb Walk.* The Gluten Co., Inc.

Mowrey, Daniel B., Ph.D. *The Scientific Validation of Herbal Medicine,* Comporant Books.

Pedersen, Mark. *Nutritional Herbology.* Pedersen Publishing.

Shook, Dr. Edward. *Beginning Treatise in Herbology. Advanced Treatise in Herbology.* Trinity Press.

Tenney, Louise, M.H. *Modern Day Plagues.*

Thakkur, Dr. Chandrashekhar. *AyurVeda.* Ancient Wisdom Publications.

Tierra, Michael. *Planetary Herbology.* Lotus Press.

Treben, Maria. *Health through God's Pharmacy. Health from God's Garden.* Wilhelm Ennsthalen Steyr (Austria).

Weed, Susan. *The Wise Woman Herbal for the Childbearing Year.* Ash Tree.

Weiner, Dr. Michael. *Weiner's Herbal.* Scarborough.

P.O. Box 412 · Springville, Utah 84663 · 1-888-489-0155 ·
www.christopherpublications.com